D1826247

POWERFUL HABITS FOR WEIGHT LOSS

SIMPLE DAILY HABITS TO LOSE WEIGHT WITHOUT DIETING.

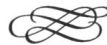

TAYLOR MACY

CONTENTS

INTRODUCTION

The year is coming to an end. Everywhere you turn, people are making plans for the new year ahead. One thing you are sure of is that you will come across many people planning to go on a diet. You have probably done it, too. Everyone has a different reason to start a diet. There are so many diets out there. Some are too fancy to be accurate, yet people still follow them. Dieting, for many people, feels like the best way to get around their weight problems. However, does it really work? Is it really a good idea to go on a diet?

Diets get a lot of publicity, and perhaps that's all they should get. You push your limits when you are on a diet. You eat food that has been specifically mapped out for you, some of which might be too expensive for you to sustain on your current budget for the long term. At times you have to stay hungry for a very long time, which might be dangerous, and could result in an eating disorder.

The problem with diets is that most of the time, the results are not sustainable. You will find a lot of information about a given diet: how it works, what you should do, and the results you should expect in a specific number of days or weeks. However, they fail to disclose the caveat that the results will not last if you stop following the diet. Many diets are only suitable for the short-term because, in order for them to work, you have to deny your body specific nutrients, which is not advisable in the long run. Going on a diet is not the right way to lose weight. So, what should you do? What is the best way to lose weight and keep it off?

Think about it; you gain weight gradually. No one goes to sleep and wakes up many pounds heavier. It all happens over time. This is one of the reasons why dieting will not work for you. Your approach to losing weight should be as gradual as you gained it. There are small changes that you can make in your lifestyle that will go a long way towards helping you lose weight. The secret lies in the things that you do every single day.

What might seem like a small change in your routine can go a long way to creating reliable results in the future. Because you will not be depriving your body of useful nutrients, your body will quickly adapt to the changes you make, and your weight loss program will be a success.

Weight loss gains should be sustainable. There is no point in losing weight if you will gain it back in a few months. Going back and forth is frustrating and sets you up for failure. You need a different approach. Think of weight gain in terms of behavioral change. Changing your mindset and behavior helps you look at weight loss from a different perspective.

You will learn how to be aware of what your body needs and what it wants. Telling the difference between these two might be the change you need in your life. You will learn that you do not always have to respond to your cravings. Cravings can mess up your weight loss plan and lead you down the path of unhealthy eating patterns that can destroy your life.

The journey to becoming self-aware is such an uplifting experience. You'll know when you are hungry and how much food is enough for you. You will learn how to identify the right ingredients when you are out shopping. These are some of those small changes you make that can have profound effects on your life.

It is easy to read success stories and imagine that the weight loss regime will be a walk in the park – this is far from reality. Considering that it is easier to gain weight than to lose it, prepare yourself for a difficult journey. You need to have a positive support system surrounding you. Ensure that your partner, family, and close friends are aware of the journey you are on so that they can support you in any way possible. There may be times when you might feel like quitting, but your support network will help you stay on course.

The lessons you learn in this book are not just about weight loss and living a healthy life. You will also learn how to translate a healthy lifestyle into a fulfilling and satisfying life. Happiness is so elusive for many people these days. This is because we pursue different illusions of happiness to the point that we forget what we actually want, and what true happiness is about. Your commitment and resilience are the keys to achieving success in your plan.

Unlike the short-term benefits of dieting, habit changes deliver long-term benefits that offer the promise of a healthy life. When you include your loved ones in your plan, they share in this amazing journey and experience, too. As they have motivated you in your quest to improve your life, so will your success motivate them to emulate you and embrace a similar method. It is so gratifying when your loved ones see you as the embodiment of success, commitment, and healthy living.

As you read this book, remember in the back of your mind that you are in charge. You have your future in the palms of your hands. Everything you desire is on the other side of fear. Diets might have let you down before, but this plan will not. This plan is not about denying yourself essential nutrients; it is about making subtle changes in your life that will make you happy for a long time. This plan is about helping you realize that you have what it takes to be the best version of yourself.

What else are you waiting for? Get up and start today! Today is just the beginning of many new journeys in the future. This is the day you begin the journey to unlock new levels of satisfaction, pleasure, healthy living, and social connections. This is the plan that will change your life!

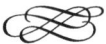

CHAPTER 1

NEGATIVE CONSEQUENCES OF DIETING

The word diet appears in conversations all the time, and its meaning can be varied. Diet can refer to a cultural food or drink that someone does or does not consume out of customary obligation, which, in essence, defines a meal plan. For example, Muslims do not eat pork due to religious restrictions. Therefore, in a Muslim household, pork does not feature in their diets at all. Diets can also be prescribed for individuals out of medical concern, like the DASH diet, which helps in controlling diabetes. The examples above depict diets whose concepts are religiously, culturally, or medically enforced, and have no direct goal of weight loss.

Other than reasons like those mentioned above, diet is commonly used in the weight watching realm. Most of the time, when discussions about diets come up, they are about individuals trying to lose weight. Most, if not all, of these diets, are restrictive in a way so that the participant can lose weight.

Reasons Why Diets Do Not Work

Diets can be harmful. They do more harm than any

benefit they bring and only provide you with temporary satisfaction. The problem with temporary satisfaction is that it breeds disappointment and frustration when you return to your original state. Many people have developed anxiety and depression because they are frustrated with their weight (Jacka & Berk, 2013). All this comes from a notion they had that they need to look a certain way, so they must eat a certain way too.

Many experts today advise their patients against dieting (Selig, 2010). Diets do not work. The damning statistics against dieting show that more than 90% of those who participate in any weight loss diet regain the weight in less than five years. This also means that you risk not only getting back that weight but getting back more than you lost. Essentially, dieting is bad for you.

But why does this happen? Let's look at the rudimentary concept of a diet. A diet is a temporary plan (Tamarkin, 2018). This simple concept is what most people ignore. They use short-term gains to support a fallacy in their minds that the results are long term. In essence, when you buy into such an idea, you only succeed at one thing – conning yourself!

The human body is built in such a way that it has a natural response mechanism for everything (Aamodt, 2013). Imagine having to remember to breathe – a lot of people would be dead because they got carried away with something, and forgot that they need to keep breathing. The body's response to hunger is one of those autonomous processes that goes on subconsciously. You do not know it happens, but it is happening, and you will end up doing something about it.

When you are hungry, your body sends signals to your brain that you need to eat. Logically, and out of necessity, you look for something to eat. When you are starving, your body is aware and goes into starvation mode, where it hoards resources to help you survive the period of scarce food. The body does this to protect you from starving.

What most diets essentially do is to starve you. In response, your body will slow down your metabolism. A slow metabolic rate means that you are sluggish in almost everything you do. In your mind, however, you think the diet is working when, in a real sense, it is not. You are just post-poning the inevitable.

The Weight Cycling Problem

Going on a diet is one of the worst mistakes you can make for one simple reason – you deprive yourself of essen-tial nutrients. There is a reason why your body needs specific nutrients. Nutrients that aid in growth, development, and nourishment. Why would you believe that something that denies you essential nutrients is good for your health? This idea alone goes against everything you might have learned about healthy eating since you were a child.

These diets trick the body into shedding weight by removing an important nutrient from your meal plan. Once you get through the "ideal" duration of the diet, your body gets back into its natural habits. For you to maintain the weight loss, you must keep eating non-nutritious meal plans all the time. This is not sustainable and is honestly an unhealthy habit.

When you get back to your regular eating habits, the weight you lost comes back, and possibly even more. This is the moment you introduce **yo-yo dieting** (weight cycling) into your life. Yo-yo dieting is a short-term cycle that bears short-term results. You are going about this the wrong way if you plan on long-term results. The only thing you will achieve is compounded disappointment.

First off, weight cycling is not good for your heart. Anything that is bad for your heart will inevitably be detri-mental to your overall health and mortality. Many people choose a specific diet, but they barely last a few days before they revert to their regular eating habits. Before you know it, you are unhappy with your weight, and you try the diet again, or another plan altogether, hoping for different results. You end up in a vicious cycle that slowly erodes your will to eat healthy. This cycle also stresses your cardiovascular system (Strohacker, Carpenter, & McFarlin, 2009).

Dysfunctional Gut

There are trillions of microbial cells in the gut. All these cells have specific roles to play, and they influence many things, including nutrition and metabolism. In a state of balance, the microbial cells perform their duties amicably. However, constant fluctuation, which yo-yo dieting causes, disrupts their normal behavior. This disruption might be responsible for conditions such as inflammatory bowel disease, and, in some people, obesity.

Promotional Wording

Take your time and review all the diets you come across online. The wording around them is all about convincing you to join. If something were that good, it would not need all the promotional verbiage. Some of the words used to promote diets include detox, cleanse, fast fat burn, guaranteed weight loss, and so forth. The list is endless.

The funny thing is, your body can do all that. It does it all the time. Your liver, if healthy, is adequately suited to detoxify the body. Your intestines do a good job, too. Why do you need to go on a diet? A diet will not accomplish all that they say it will. Your body organs do their work. The diet sensationalizes the concept of what you are looking for.

Another concept that is often passed along with diets is *fast and easy*. In this life, nothing worthwhile comes that quickly and easily. Everything about honest success comes gradually as you lay credible foundations. Do you know that there are dangers associated with rapid fat loss? Burning fat too quickly can lead to ketosis (Gao, et al., 2017). Ketosis refers to an unhealthy buildup of urine and ketones in the blood, which is toxic. Another problem with rapid weight loss is that the body has to draw energy from your lean muscles. Therefore, your muscles must work harder to burn energy, weakening them over time. Before you know it, you are lethargic and can barely get through a hectic day.

Forget about the miracles that diets promise you. None of this is true. What benefit is short-term gratification to you, when it comes at the expense of your long-term satisfaction? When the diet runs its course, and you get back to your regular eating habits, you will pack on some weight. At this point, you will blame yourself and feel terrible about your life choices. This causes further problems in your life as shame, self-doubt, and depression set in. In your desire to feel better and prove yourself and everyone else wrong, you find another diet, and the vicious cycle continues.

Yo-Yo Dieting

The simplest definition of yo-yo dieting is a procedure where you lose weight, gain it, then go on a diet to lose weight again. It is a cycle, one that you need to stop. It is called yo-yo dieting because your weight is always up and down like a yo-yo. It is one of the most common predicaments today, yet the dangers associated with it are mind-boggling. A practice that you embrace to suit your lifestyle eventually becomes the source of your downfall. Here are some reasons why you need to stop yo-yo dieting:

• **Guaranteed Weight Gain** — In your pursuit of weight loss, the yo-yo mechanism is a sure guarantee that you will gain weight in the long run, defeating the purpose. The role of the leptin hormone is to signal the body that you are full, so you can stop eating. In the course of a diet, fat loss means the body's production of leptin is reduced. Usually, when the body releases leptin into the bloodstream, you are signaled to eat less because you already have energy stores. When you lose weight drastically, the production of leptin decreases while your appetite hits the roof (Considine, 2003). At this point, your body is trying to stockpile and replenish your energy supply. Your body will conserve energy to make up for the muscle mass you lost while dieting. It is quite unfortunate that, at the end of a diet, most people will regain up to 65% of the weight they lost within a year, and a third of people who use diets become heavier than they were when they started. If you believe in diets, this *up* phase of your yo-yo cycle will prompt you to find another diet, so you lose weight.

• **Muscle Loss** — On a weight loss diet, your body will lose body fat and muscle mass. You can regain fat faster than muscle after losing weight. Therefore, the longer you stay on a weight loss diet, the higher your risk of muscle loss, which will also affect your physical strength.

• **Limited Prospects for the Future** — Diets focus on short-term gains. This explains why they are often endorsed by celebrities. Celebrities live a different lifestyle than you do. They often have a few weeks to get in shape to suit a specific role for the film they are shooting. Once the film is over, they work their way back to normal meals. The problem with these diets is that they encourage you to follow a given set of rules up to a certain point in time when your goals have been met. What happens after that? How do you move on from the diet back to your normal life? This lack of integration makes it impossible for you to experience long-term weight loss benefits.

• **Disappointment and Frustration** — You put a lot of work, determination, and sacrifice into diets that you hope will work out in the long run. However, this never happens. One moment you are enjoying some fantastic results, and a few weeks later you are heavier than you have ever been. If you do these two or three times, it will inevitably become frustrating at some point. People who have been through this do not only feel frustrated, they are not happy about their health, and their lives in general. This also affects your confidence and self-esteem (Son & Kim, 2012).

- **Risk of Heart Disease** — Yo-yo dieting is not just unhealthy; it also leaves your heart at risk. People who stick to these regimes are at risk of developing coronary artery disease. Coronary artery disease is a condition where the heart-supplying arteries become narrower (Grady, 2004). While being overweight increases your risk of heart disease, weight gain is worse. The on and off nature of weight cycling will further worsen your predicament. The yo-yo effect of gaining weight after you stop dieting can also increase your blood pressure. If you maintain a weight cycling regime, your body gets conditioned to accept specific changes, which makes it difficult for you to stabilize your blood pressure in the future after weight loss.

- **Risk of Diabetes** — Weight cycling is one of the risk factors for developing type 2 diabetes. At the end of these diets, most people gain weight in the form of belly fat. You have a higher chance of developing diabetes from belly fat than fat stored in other parts of the body, like your hips, legs, or arms. Your body will produce insulin in large quantities to try and handle the situation. Increased insulin in the blood is one of the earliest signs that you might have diabetes.

- **Fatty Liver** — A fatty liver is a situation where your body has too much fat and stores some of it in the liver. When this happens, you are at risk of becoming obese and developing diabetes. There is also a likelihood that you might develop liver cirrhosis. If you consistently go on weight cycling diets, things could get out of hand very fast.

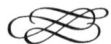

CHAPTER 2

CHANGE YOUR MINDSET TO CHANGE YOUR BODY

*W*hat is your definition of failure, and do you believe you have ever failed in life? Failure is not tangible. It is a belief. Core beliefs are ideologies you hold in high regard, and that define your life. They are the ideas that make your life what it is today. In a way, beliefs give your life structure. There are things you can do and others you avoid altogether because you grew up believing that they are not right.

Many patients who have succeeded in therapy did so because they learned how to reframe their thoughts. When you have a negative view of your life, it is impossible to see anything positive about it, even if everyone else sees it. Your idea of positivity is that it will not last. You get used to negative vibes to the point where positivity is nothing but a fallacy in your life.

Your mindset is a culmination of notations, methods, and assumptions (Issler, 2009). The mindset is a very powerful tool because it is set in your subconscious mind. The subconscious mind gets you in a routine; you will do things not because you have to or need to, but because your body knows no other way.

The power of your mindset is so incredible that it influences your decisions (Oppong, 2018). You might not know outright why you have a predisposition to certain people. Your subconscious mind with its core beliefs, however, finds some similarities in the way these people go about their lives. As a result, you find yourself drawn to them, and will follow them anywhere without batting an eyelid.

What does your body have to do with your mindset? Your mindset determines your perception of success, failure, and happiness (Hildrew, 2018). You have specific body goals that you must achieve in order to be content. To meet these goals, your mindset and your desire must be aligned. Without that, your efforts will be futile. The following are some simple yet effective ways you can change your mindset and induce the changes you want to see in yourself:

• **Identify Your Mindset** — You cannot change what you don't know. The first step toward success is to identify what you want to change. Think about your goals, then ask yourself what is holding you back from achieving them. Think about your current mindset. Do you feel that the things you believe are useful and support your long-term goals? If you have some roadblocks or obstacles, get rid of them. Anything that holds you back embeds deep within your subconscious.

People who live healthy lives generally have a tendency to eat healthy food, exercise often, and generally take care of their bodies. When they are out eating, it is not just about satisfaction, but about what they are introducing to their body. They think about the long-term effects of the food they eat. You need to become aware of what you are eating and why. When you embrace the mentality of a healthy individual, you are helping your brain recreate and embrace a new concept of healthy living. Do not force yourself to do this. You need to enjoy this and want it for yourself. Your mind is more receptive to things that are pleasurable to you. If you love the new changes towards living a healthy life, you look forward to them and become more positive about your life. You need to first identify as somebody that eats healthy, even though you might have a long history of eating poorly. When you make that mental adjustment that you are no longer that person, that you are now somebody that eats healthy, all of your actions will start to fall into place.

If you identify as somebody that is trying to lose weight, that isn't a commitment. That is a weak mindset and one that is easy to break. You need to break away from your old self, with your old habits and the only way to do that is to identify with a new vision and outlook on life. When you see somebody that is in shape, they most likely identify as somebody that eats healthy, and they embody that lifestyle. If that same person were to identify as somebody that is lazy and eat anything in front of them, pretty soon, they would experience rapid weight gain, and they will no longer feel fit. It is a mental shift that will direct the body and the habits you form. It all starts with your mindset!

• **Search for Useful Information** — Always try to find credible information about the things you want to change in your life. Today, we are lucky to have a wealth of information on the Internet.

One of the biggest mistakes most people make is that they do not go out of their way to look for information. The few people who look for information do not investigate their sources carefully, and, as a result, they end up with everything but useful and accurate information. Take some time and read useful, credible material about the subject of your mindset change. Informational articles and journals are incredibly useful in this regard. Try to avoid public discussion forums. Most forums are full of speculation, biased information, and promotional pieces that might leave you more confused than when you started.

- **Change Your Language** — What words do you use to speak to yourself? Many people who use defeatist words never succeed. If you tell yourself that you will never be good enough, your mind registers this, and it becomes the norm.

Whenever you face a challenge, your immediate response will be that you are not good enough. With that in mind, you barely pull your weight. Changing your mindset involves changing the way you speak to yourself about the things you can do and the things you cannot. You are challenging yourself to become a better person. There is no room for negativity or self-deprecation here. Try to remind yourself of all the good things that are going on in your life. Encourage yourself to learn from them and build from there. Everyone has problems or challenges they are struggling to overcome. Do not dwell on them. What you are trying to do is create an enabling environment of abundance rather than strife and fear in your mind.

- **Embrace Healthy Self-Motivation** — Self-motivation helps you create a positive attitude that leads to results. With this mindset, nothing can stand in your way. You believe in the change you want, and more importantly, you believe in the process. Negative self-talk holds many people back. Instead, try to empower yourself. Remind yourself that you are good enough, and there are many awesome rewards ahead. Change is never easy, so it is important to stay positive. This is a journey, and it is incredibly rewarding!

- **Leave Your Comfort Zone** — Stepping out of your comfort zone is not easy if you do not realize you are in one. Comfort zones create an illusion that you have made it in life, and everything is okay. It gets worse when you settle into a comfort zone when things are going well. Very soon, you forget about your struggles, your efforts, and every other obstacle you had to overcome to be where you are. Challenge yourself to be better to improve. Challenges encourage you to rise to the occasion.

Think of yourself as a popular smartphone app. While the app is amazing and has millions of active users, upgrades and updates are necessary from time to time. Security patches keep the app users safe from attacks and harmful exploits. Updating the app refines it and makes the user experience better. Updates are a necessity if the app is to stay ahead of the game for a long time. The same applies to your life. Do things that will make you a better person. This doesn't mean you should not enjoy your success. Embrace it, appreciate it, and move on. Challenging yourself to step out of a comfort zone is a good way to create an environment where your brain is always proactive.

- **Make Habitual Changes** — Changing your mindset requires habitual changes, too. Try to introduce some activities into your plan that help to reinforce what you are working towards. If you are working towards a growth mindset from a fixed perspective, for example, you must create some room for learning. Believe in the fact that the changes you make are a journey, not a destination. There will be many lessons along the way. Note them as you go. Use them as empowering tools to help you create an environment of success.
- **Build a Healthy Support Network** — The people around you have a more significant hold on your life than you may realize. As we mentioned earlier on, you are drawn to some people because of your subconscious belief that your ideologies are aligned. If you want to change your life, spend more time with people who are on the same path. This way, you can learn from them as they will from you. It is always easier to embrace a new mindset when you can see people around you, striving for the same thing. When you see how

their lives are improving, it is easier for you to adapt and change the way you go about your life to match your mindset.

Creating a Vision for Success

One of the most important lessons you will learn in life is to envision your success. If you can dream it, you can live it. While this might sound corny, there are very real benefits of going through this exercise. Creating a vision elevates your ideas beyond the ordinary. There are many things you wish you could achieve, but somehow, you never seem to have time for them. It is overwhelming when you think about all the things you pushed to the back of your list of priorities and forgot about. Think of all of the New Year's resolutions that were brushed aside after March.

Fear causes paralysis. Most of the time, we worry about the things we cannot do, instead of those we can do. If you have a vision, you can overcome this problem. A vision gives you a way to remind yourself of why you are working so hard. It helps you understand your plans and stay positive and focused on your goals. More importantly, visions strengthen your belief in yourself (Hathaway, 2017).

A vision for success is like a mirage. You have a picture of it in your mind and would love to see it manifest in the real world. Each time you recall this image, it grows into an idea that evolves into a conception, something your subconscious wills into existence. Visions are about expecting the future to be better than your present, and working towards achieving it.

Visions are important because each decision we make in life comes with consequences. Without a vision, you will struggle to live the life you desire or deserve. Visions strengthen your resolve. The stronger and more realistic your visions are, the easier it is for you to establish and live a balanced life.

When you think about your visions, think about empowering your inner-self. Your visions should give you purpose, satisfaction, and fulfillment. They bring meaning into your life, especially when your visions connect with your deeper needs and desires.

At first, your vision might feel like a jigsaw puzzle with a hundred thousand pieces scattered all over. You struggle to imagine where to begin. However, when you are calm and collected, you figure out a way to put the pieces together. How do you turn those amazing ideas into reality? The following ideas will guide you and help you stay sharp and focused on your vision:

- **What is Truly Important To You?** — What do you really want? This is an important question that many people can barely answer. What matters most to you gives you purpose. If you 'kinda' want something you are not likely willing to sacrifice for it. If you have a passion for something, then you will have the internal motivation to help you achieve that outcome.

Your visions are empty without purpose. They are things you feel so deeply about that you cannot logically explain them to someone. You either feel them, or you don't. Taking this approach to your vision will help you figure out what is most important to you. Then, you can iron out the process of getting there. You bought this book, that is a first step towards achieving your goal of losing weight and having sustained success. The vision you have of yourself will help guide you when you are having to make those tough decisions of sticking to your healthy eating habits.

- **Make Time for Planning** — All great accomplishments take time and planning. Anyone who tries to convince you they succeeded overnight is not being totally honest. In your vision for success, there should be room for planning. Have a list of things you need to achieve. Organize the list into priorities.

The beauty of planning is that it does not take a lot of your time. Write down these goals and make them real. You need to write down ideas for your vision. This way, you have a reference point. A reference point helps you evaluate your performance in terms of achieving your goals. Ask yourself what you have achieved so far. Compare that with what you achieved in the previous evaluation period. When you do this, you can track your progress and identify where you need to buckle down and put in more effort. Remember that setting goals should always be an ongoing process. You refine the process over time with each milestone to achieve the best results. Revisit these goals often to make sure you stay on track.

Some examples might be:
- What is your goal weight?
- What is your goal clothing size?
- What date do you wish to achieve that weight?
- What milestones along the way should you track?

• **Embrace the Results** — The results you derive from your vision for success are a product of all the effort you put into the process. You are changing your reality one step at a time. There might be some uncertainty as you proceed with your plans, but that should not hold you back. You should embrace the results you get, celebrate them, and improve on the areas you need to. This is how the long game is played. You make adjustments to a working formula and improve on the next evaluation period.

How to Overcome Limiting Beliefs

It is easy for us to be victims of our own limiting beliefs. If we have struggled with weight in the past, these are the only reference points our mind has to reflect upon. Many times we have tried and failed at losing weight. Or maybe if we did lose weight, we weren't able to maintain that success, and we gained it all back. Failure after failure compound in our minds, and it starts to spread into other areas of our life. Limiting beliefs are dangerous and something that we need to address and overcome. If you can overcome your limiting beliefs, you are opening yourself up for new possibilities. Some of the greatest men and women in history had also had to overcome their own limiting beliefs when they faced adversity. When we are discussing some of the greatest minds and inventors of all time, the list is never complete without Thomas Edison. After all, it was through his work that many modern-day technological developments were born. By the time of his death in 1931, Edison had more than a thousand patents in the US alone (Edison, 1900).

Edison did not immediately succeed; he failed many times before he succeeded in his attempts. But we do not remember Edison's failures, we remember him for his many successes. Many years later, motivational speakers still use some of his quotes as inspiration to encourage their audiences never to give up. Things will not always go your way, but that does not mean that you should quit. There are always lessons in failure, lessons that can make you a better person, and eventually make success sweeter than you had imagined.

Picture Edison, whose teacher was constantly frustrated and impatient with him, turning out to be one of the most prolific inventors in history. What if he had taken his teacher's words to heart and given up on learning? Life would have taken an unprecedented turn. In his first attempts in the employment industry, he was fired because he was not productive, yet he still did not give up.

Believe in yourself. Focus on something you want and go for it. Do not let anything hold you back. It has been said before that Edison failed a thousand times before he perfected the light bulb. Different sources quote different figures. However, the lesson is not about the number of times he failed, but about his persistence.

Changing your mindset will not always be a smooth journey. Things will go wrong from time to time, and this is normal. In life, things do not always go according to plan. Your desire, passion, and resolve for success, however, should never change. You might be your own worst enemy or your greatest ally. Each morning when you look in the mirror, the face that looks back at you is the only person standing in your way. You can conquer everything and everyone else, but if you are unable to believe in yourself, you will never truly appreciate what you have become.

There will be slip ups and setbacks. Eating healthy is something you strive for as a goal, not something that you will achieve every single day. If you overindulge, don't get frustrated and give up on your goals. Reset, and start over with your next meal. That's the beauty of eating healthy and implementing good habits. You have so many opportunities to succeed. Each meal is a new opportunity.

Success is not easy to achieve, but failure hurts more, especially when you realize how much you would have achieved if you had never given up.

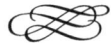

CHAPTER 3

THE POWER OF CREATING HABITS

*E*veryone has some habits that they cannot drop. Some are good, and others are bad. Habits influence everything you do (Nöth, 2016). Some of the things you do out of habit have become so routine that you cannot even explain why you do them. Perhaps the closest explanation is that, to you, it is common sense to do them. In fact, you often assume that everyone else does it the way you do. You find it difficult to understand how someone gets on with his or her life without following the same patterns that you do. Some habits might be completely foreign to you in the beginning. The habits of somebody that is in great shape are most likely completely different than the habits of somebody that is obese.

You don't have to think hard to conceptualize a habit. Start from the time you wake up. Today, most people reach for their phones to check and clear notifications. Some people make a beeline for the bathroom when they wake up to freshen up and begin their day. Even the route you use to school or work is the same unless there's major traffic or an accident.

Habits are deliberate choices that the brain makes. It is really all about conditioning (Verplanken & Aarts, 1999). When you are young, you have to learn everything. However, you learn to do things a certain way, and it remains in your subconscious. Your mind creates a new reality each time you perform some repetitive tasks, and they become habits.

When you move to a new town, everything you knew about your former town makes it difficult for you to adjust and adapt. You struggle to find your way around town; you cannot enjoy the restaurants yet, and so forth. After a while, your brain accepts the fact that things have changed, and you need to learn how to do things differently in order to survive in this new place. This is the point at which you start embracing your new environment and find your place in it.

The human body is a self-sufficient one. Your body is always looking for ways to make your life easier. Your brain remembers the things you frequently do, and after some time, they become habits you perform automatically. Think of your brain like a web browser. Each time you visit a website, your browser stores some files in the background in the form of cookies. This is called caching. A browser cache makes your work easier because, each time you visit the website, your browser remembers that you have been there before. It does not have to load photos, videos, and other content again, which consumes a lot of time and bandwidth. Your browser simply checks its memory and retrieves the information you need. If you frequent the website, it also updates the content in its memory so that you are always accessing the most recent version of the website. This is exactly what your brain does when you form habits.

Distinct Features of a Habit

The brain identifies and creates a habit in a three-step plan that involves cues, routines, and rewards (Orbell & Verplanken, 2010). Cues are the triggers your brain recog-

19

nizes to choose the right habit to initiate. Routines refer to the manner in which habits influence your thoughts, feelings, and actions. Rewards are unique grading systems your brain uses to assign value to habits. The brain also uses rewards to determine whether to remember or drop a habit (Bokhari).

Say you plan to create a habit where you go jogging every day after work. How do you go about it? First, you need to choose the right cue. Keep your running shoes in your car. You want to develop a routine of running 3 miles after work. Each time you leave work and see the shoes, your brain reminds you that it's time to change into your running attire and head to the park or gym.

At the end of every run, perhaps you get a healthy smoothie. This is your reward. Each time you think about a vegetable smoothie, your brain reminds you that you should get to the park for your 3-mile run. In this case, craving a smoothie becomes the difference between going for a run or not.

Cravings can influence habits, and habits can powerfully induce neurological cravings. Identifying what induces your cravings is the first step towards understanding your habits.

How Do Habits Influence Your Life?

As we have seen above, habits make your work easier. You don't have to think about some things. Your brain picks up on some cues, and you automatically know what to do. For example, you don't have to remember to take a shower in the morning. You know that, before you get dressed and go to work, you must shower. This is something you do without even thinking about it. You are on autopilot.

Habits have a significant influence on our lives. The majority of the things we do every day are out of habit. You might think that you made a conscious decision to do something, but in reality, your brain just prefers it because you are used to it. This also means that you can change your behavior by understanding and changing some habits. Do you think you made a decision to brush your teeth before you go to bed, or was it a habit that was instilled in you at a young age?

Habits are not set in stone. They are flexible and can change according to your immediate needs in the current environment. With the right stimuli, you can drop a habit and pick an alternative one that makes you feel better. At times, all you need to do is change your routine, and you can drop an old or bad habit.

There is a ripple effect in small wins that impacts different spheres of your life. Small wins give you a winning platform upon which you can build for the future. You are more confident about your life and activities, and you want to carry on winning. Besides, winning is addictive. If you start working out more often, you will start eating healthier food, too. These two go hand in hand because you want to keep enjoying and maximizing the benefits. The next time you reach for the ice cream, you will remember the hard work you put in already, and it will motivate you to stay on track. Success leads to more success.

Your brain does not need your permission to form a habit ("Charles Duhigg's 'The Power of Habit' - 13 Key Insights", 2015). It identifies cues, links the triggers to a routine, and anticipates a reward. All of this happens without your knowledge. Each time you think about the reward, it creates a craving that needs to be acted upon. Your brain then directs you to do something out of habit. If you love the rewards, your brain is impressed, and that particular habit loop is appreciated. The trick is to make sure you are properly rewarding yourself for the habit you are creating. Only you know what works for you. This goes back to taking the time to put a proper plan in place.

You will need to train your willpower in order to see

success. Training is not just about your muscles and losing weight. You can also train your willpower. You have a lot to do during the day, and this can be exhausting. When you are almost giving up, you push yourself more until you accomplish your goals, and your willpower can get exhausted. In other words, you feel burned out. When this happens, you fall into old habits like eating junk food. Remind yourself that you are stronger, and focus on the greater objective, losing weight. This is not something that will come easily. This takes time, and you will fail many times starting out. Don't feel discouraged. Every day is a new opportunity to succeed. That is why it is so important to have a clear vision for success. If you know where you want to be, you will be able to pick yourself back up when you stumble.

Why Are Habits Important?

A healthy lifestyle is the sum of many activities, including healthy eating, exercise, and other activities that eventually become regular habits. Nearly everyone in a position of authority will, at some point in time, encourage you to form good habits. From life coaches to your teachers, parents, colleagues, and doctors, they all insist you need to get into the habit of doing something positive. Have you ever wondered why habits are this important?

Habits are important because they are a reflection of who you are (Kim, 2015). These are activities you perform daily without thinking about them. Since they become your routine, they become an embodiment of the person you are. For example, when law enforcement officers are looking for an elusive criminal, they study his habits and lay traps for him. This technique works because, by studying the criminal's habits, they can predict his next move. They might not know the criminal in person, but knowledge of his habits helps them create a persona that they can understand in order to track and catch that criminal. Along those same lines, if you were to list out all of your daily habits on a piece of paper, would they represent that habits of somebody living a healthy lifestyle or would they represent the habits of somebody that was overweight and unmotivated. You are the sum of your habits. Take a moment to reflect on your daily routines. I like to create a T chart and list my positive habits on the left side and my negative habits on the right side. This is a tough exercise and one that requires you to be brutally honest with yourself. Find ways to reinforce your good habits. Also, find ways to replace your bad habits.

Another reason why habits are important is because they are flexible. You can change habits that do not suit you or your plans. It is difficult to drop old habits, but it is not impossible. It just takes a stronger resolve. All you need to do is make a small change in your life and stick to it until it becomes a routine. This goes back to your vision and the life you want to create for yourself. Stay disciplined when you want to continue with your bad habit. Remind yourself that you are working towards a goal. Reward yourself when you do something other than the bad habit. This sends positive reinforcement back to your brain.

Marathon runners do not wake up one day and sign up for a marathon without ever having run before. They prepare for months or years before they are ready to compete. Creating a daily habit like training will get them to the final lap of the race. If you feel that you could use a better job than what you currently have, you start by actively searching for one. Habits, therefore, play an important role in goal setting. I remember the first time I ever ran a half marathon. I HATE running. I knew there was no way on earth I would ever be able to finish 13.1 miles. But I knew I could run one mile. And so I did. Then I ran 2 miles. Then after a while, I ran 3. I would push myself and then reset my goals. Eventually, I was up to 10 miles. It wasn't all at once; it took months. If I had tried to run all 13.1 miles on my first day, I would have fallen over and given up. It is great you are reading this book, but there is no way you are going to be able to incorporate all of the habits all at once. You need to set goals, and then once you achieve them, reward yourself and then recalibrate to push yourself out of your comfort zone once again. Really push yourself so that over time you become the best version of yourself. I know this can be very difficult because it is so easy to be motivated when you read this text or listen to a podcast about achieving our goal, but the real work takes place when you are forced to make those tough decisions. That's why creating habits are so important. It takes the decision making out of the equation and becomes something that you do. But that also takes time, so you start that process by setting goals, and soon you will be on your way.

Do you have life goals that you hope to achieve someday? The idea of the goal alone will not help you achieve your dreams. You must form a habit of working towards that goal. Based on the size of your life plan, you can break it into smaller plans that you can accomplish in phases as you work towards the greater plan.

It is easy to waste time on unnecessary activities or spend more time than you need on something important. Many people would jump at the idea of not doing anything challenging at all. Creating good habits helps you learn to manage your time, be more efficient, and end up with more time to rest. This really comes into play when it involves cooking healthy meals. It is much easier to swing by the local fast food and pick up something because that takes less time. If you properly manage your time, you can avoid these traps. One of the best ways of doing this is to meal prep, which we will talk more about later.

There will be days when you won't feel like working on

anything at all. This lack of motivation plagues everyone at some point. Perhaps you don't feel like eating healthy, working out, or going out of the house. I know that feeling all too well. I will throw on Netflix, pull out my smartphone, and order something from Postmates or UberEats. Sounds like a relaxing Sunday but the problem with that is that it doesn't get you closer to your goal and doesn't align with the vision that you have set for yourself.

That doesn't mean you can't enjoy a day of relaxation. Motivation can dissipate in response to different stimuli, events, and activities in your life. If you create a habit of doing things, you will get through them whether you are motivated or not. You know you must do it, so nothing else matters. It is just one thing you have to check off of your list for the day. Rather than wasting your day, if you have formed the habit of running 3 miles, you will feel the need to get up off the couch and exercise before you relax. You will enjoy that movie so much more knowing that you are relaxing guilt-free because you have already completed your cardio for the day.

Benefits of Healthy Habits

Healthy habits go a long way. A healthy habit refers to any activity or behavior that has a positive effect on your emotional, mental, and physical health. Such habits have you feeling good about your life, and improve your well-being.

Given the kind of lifestyle choices that many of us make today, healthy habits are not easy to develop. You must change your mindset in order to embrace some of these changes. Once you are willing to give up some bad habits, you can look forward to amazing benefits in return, irrespective of your age or level of physical activity. The following are some of the benefits of practicing healthy lifestyle habits:

- **Weight Management** — When you get into the habit of

working out regularly and eating right, you will avoid adding weight. Once you attain your ideal weight, you can maintain it easily, too. Physical activity is important in any weight management plan. Even if your plan is not to lose weight, frequent exercise will help you stay healthy by improving your heart health, increasing your energy level, and supporting your immune system.

- **More Energy** – Regular exercise is directly correlated with the amount of energy you will have throughout the day. When you are eating healthy and exercising regularly, your body will reward you with an endless supply of energy, so you are firing on all cylinders throughout the day. I will warn you, if you are not exercising regularly and you decide to start working out, you will feel drained in the beginning, it is totally natural. Your body is not used to you expending all of this energy, and your metabolism will take some time to catch up. Do not fear, it will catch up, and the results are amazing! Another reason why habits are so powerful and help you shift your focus from short term results into long term success.

- **Lightens Your Mood** — Your body and mind are interconnected. Every good thing you do for your body eventually pays off for your mind, too. Physical activities trigger your body to produce endorphins. These are the chemicals responsible for feelings of relaxation and happiness. A healthy diet alongside physical activity will help you maintain an amazing physique, which has a positive impact on your self-esteem and confidence. Happier moods are not only connected to healthy eating and exercise. Forging healthy social connections is another habit that will increase your happiness. Fulfilling social interactions can make a big difference in your life. Resist the temptation to isolate yourself. Engage and spend time with your friends and family members often. Are you missing someone? Meet up with them, or if that is not possible, get on that video call and talk to them.

• **Disease Prevention** — High blood pressure, stroke, diabetes, heart disease, and cancer are some of the common killers in the world today. Many people are suffering because of the lifestyle choices they made that can be traced back to bad habits. You can avoid these by embracing some simple good habits. Essentially, do all you can to take good care of your body. This means you should eat right and exercise frequently. The immediate results here are healthy cholesterol levels and stable blood pressure. Since your blood is flowing smoothly, your risk of heart diseases is lower. The long-term impact is that you are at a lower risk of suffering any of the life-threatening conditions mentioned above. You can support this initiative by having a thorough physical examination annually. These exams help your doctor identify worrying symptoms early on, and they can advise you on important habitual changes that can get your life back on track.

• **You Are What You Eat** — Unhealthy food burdens your body. This explains why you often feel lethargic after consuming unhealthy foods, especially when you overeat. A balanced diet, on the other hand, feeds your body all the necessary nutrients, which means you have the fuel necessary to keep your energy levels stable. So, what should you include in this diet? Make sure you have a healthy choice of vegetables, fruits, low-fat dairy products, lean meats, and whole grains. If you get into the habit of regular exercise as well, your muscles will be stronger, you will be energetic, and your endurance level will improve. An energetic body will get you through the most challenging of days without feeling depleted at the end of the day.

How to Stick to Habits

By now, you understand why habits are important, and

the impact that they have on your life. You have also identified some habits that you need to change so you can reap amazing benefits in the future. The challenge is sticking to habits. How do you go about it?

You know how easy it is to start a new habit and struggle to see it through. While discipline is necessary, not everyone has the same resolve. The following are some simple ideas that can help you learn how to follow your habit:

• **Consistency** — You must be consistent in everything you do. If you want to run a marathon, you have to train daily. Consistency is THE key ingredient to long term success. If you can consistently make smart, healthy decisions, you will be amazed at your results. Friends and family will see you six months from now and be shocked at your transformation. Crash diets are great for short term change, but they lack consistency. Forming healthy habits are what is going to set you up for a lifetime of success.

• **Commitment** — On average, it takes around four weeks for your brain to form a habit. Try to hold on until your brain recognizes the habit as an automatic response to stimuli. You will appreciate the results. Having a strong vision will help you stay committed. I have felt that surge of excitement that today was going to be the day I was going to start eating healthy! It is so easy to convince ourselves that we were ready to change. Its a great feeling but it never lasted. I would wait a few hours until I become hungry again and then I would order a pizza and tell myself that I would start again tomorrow. It was always tomorrow. It wasn't until I made a commitment to myself that I was going to form healthy eating habits that began to see lasting change. It was difficult at first. Your body will fight you and make you want to fall into old routines but don't let it. You made a commitment, and you are sticking to it!

• **Simplicity** — With habits, you don't need something

complicated. You understand the triggers and rewards. All you have to do is change the routine. A simple change that delivers gigantic results is enough motivation for you to keep going. The more complicated something is, the harder it will be to stick to it. Keep things simple! I cannot stress this enough. The more complicated a routine, the less likely it will be that you stick to it. Start small and build on your success.

- **Habit Stacking** - This is a powerful technique that allows you to build off the success of one small change and grow that into a series of more complex routines. The purpose of habit-stacking is to create simple and repeatable routines. The goal is to make things so automated that you don't have to think about whether or not to perform an action. You accomplish this by doing the same set of actions in the same order and way each day. The trick to consistency is to treat a habit stack like a single action instead of a series of individual tasks. For Example, let's say you would like to start jogging in the morning, but you can't figure out why you aren't consistently doing this. Habit stacking is a great solution to get you started. When you first wake up, you might get out of bed and grab a glass of water. Since you are already in this habit, you build on that and incorporate the next habit. So the night before, you lay out your running shoes in front of the sink so that when you grab your glass of water in the morning, you are prompted to put on your running shoes. Now you are going to start taking action to run in the morning. You can build on from there until you have an entire morning routine all built from starting with a glass of water.

- **Journaling** — Journaling your habits and activities is a good way to remind yourself of what lies ahead and how to get there. It also helps you track progress, and each time you feel like giving up, you can look back at how far you have come. There are many different ways to do this, so it is important for you to find out what works best for you. I found early success using Bullet Journals to track my goals, eating patterns, weight loss, and habits. It was nice having everything in one place that I could go to, and either set my goals in the morning or review my outcomes at night. There are a lot of resources online around bullet journaling. There are also apps that you can download to track your progress. MyFitnessPal is a good one to log your emails and make sure you are sticking to your Macros. I also bought a Fitbit Aria which would track my weight and Body Mass Index every morning and log it online for me to review. This helped me stay on track and was also very simple to use. Find what works best for you and stick with it.

• **Partners in Crime** — Having someone to go through your habit change journey is one of the best decisions you will ever make. If you don't have someone close, you can find a life coach. These are people who will motivate you and remind you of what's at stake. Having somebody else hold you accountable is incredibly powerful, especially in the beginning. Whether or not they are going through the weight loss journey with you, they can help you stay on track and make sure you are implementing the healthy habits that align with your goal. Along those same lines, You are working hard to improve yourself. The habit-changing plan is not about anyone else. Disregard the naysayers. If you allow them an audience, they will succeed at making you feel guilty. Focus on what's good for you.

• **Perfect Imperfections** — If you expect everything to work out exactly the way you pictured it in your mind all the time, you should also prepare for epic disappointment. Things don't always work out. Accept the results and try something else. Stay focused on your objectives during the first four weeks. Don't change a thing. This is the experimenting period, after which you can evaluate the process and determine what to change. Keep a journal if needed ("How to Use a Bullet Journal Habit Tracker", 2019). The experiment phase is not always easy. Many things can go wrong. If you give up right now, you might never get back on the right track. Besides, experiments must always allow room for error.

- **Eliminate Temptations** — All your hard work can be ruined by something small in your home. Get rid of temptations. Remove junk from your pantry and your fridge for a start. We will discuss this further in a later section when we talk about creating an environment of success. In short, if you have unhealthy food lying around your kitchen, you will eat them. Be intentional when you grocery shop and don't be tempted to buy your favorite snacks because once you bring them home, you will eat them.

- **Remember the Pain** — There are consequences to dropping out before you complete the habit change process. Read about some of the risks involved if you don't see this through. Read about real-life experiences of people who have been through what you are going through. This should motivate you to try harder.

- **Dream About the Benefits** — You have to want the benefits of your habit change enough that it keeps you focused. Find books and other study materials that outline what lies ahead if you make it. This should also motivate you to stay strong and complete the mission.

When it comes to habits, always remember that big changes first start with small daily changes. It is these small changes in your lifestyle that eventually become the big improvements everyone notices.

People who have seen you struggle through the yo-yo effect of dieting might be surprised when you lose weight and maintain a lean body for years. They might have gotten accustomed to seeing you lose weight and grow fatter within a few months. However, when you change your perspective and learn to do things differently, the results, in the long run, will be amazing.

Another thing you must remember about this weight loss journey is that it is not easy, and it has never been. You have to be disciplined. Remember why you are making these changes in your life. If you decide to quit smoking, quit. Don't allow anyone to pressure you into going back. If you are cutting off alcohol, do it. At the end of the day, you are the only one who knows how difficult your weight struggle is, and what you are doing about it.

Healthy Activities for a Healthy Life

The following are some activities that you can engage in regularly, and that will have a profound impact on your life. Not all of the information here will be mind-blowing. A lot of it is very basic, but when compounded with other healthy habits will lead to incredible results. You can take some of these examples and find ways for you to habit stack so that it becomes part of an overall healthy routine.

• **Stand up Regularly** — Many people worry about the lack of regular exercise. We don't work out as often as we should. A new problem is arising, especially in modern work centers where people are generally immobile and sedentary. You spend many hours in the office sitting at your desk with very little movement. Such immobility impedes your body's ability to process sugars and fats, which creates even more health problems for you as they accumulate in the body. Move around the office a bit. If you need to make a call, take it on the move. Walk to your friend's office. Standing desks are a great option as well, I just installed one at my home office, and I love it! Do whatever it takes to get up and move around. Set an alarm, so you get up every hour to stretch your legs. One of the habits I implemented was drinking more water throughout the day. Because of this, I had to go to the restroom much more often. Instead of going to the restroom next to my office, I made it a point to walk to the restroom that was all the way down the hall. This was a small change, but it was easy, and I stuck to it.

• **Physical Activity** — Working your muscles has long-term benefits. As you grow older, you become vulnerable to injuries, fractures, back pain, and osteoporosis. You don't have to get to that point. Find activities that work your muscles, like hiking, yoga, walking up flights of stairs, and so on. You would be amazing at all of your day to day activities that you can incorporate. Start small and work your way up. Do you work in an office that has stairs? Great, take them! You will be amazed at how much energy you expend when you take the stairs instead of the elevator. If you are just starting out, you don't have to do it all at once. Take the stairs for the first few floors then take the elevator the rest. Do whatever works best for you as long as you are pushing yourself out of your normal sedentary habits and working towards your vision of success.

• **Find Time to be Outdoors** — Go outside and enjoy the fresh air. There are so many activities that you can engage in outdoors. I wanted to be outside more, but I didn't have anyone to go outside with me, so I decided to adopt a puppy! It was the best decision I have ever made. We regularly go for walks because I know he doesn't want to be cooped up all day in the house either. I realize adopting a puppy might not be realistic for your situation, but you can find a way to adapt to your surroundings. Go for a walk around your neighborhood. Park in the furthest parking spot when you go to the store. Any way you can add more activity to your day to day is a step in the right direction.

• **Maintain the Right Posture** — When you were young, you probably got into trouble with your teacher or your parents because you were not sitting up straight. Fixing your posture helps your body muscles work in the right way. This will also reduce joint pressure, which reduces your vulnerability to back pain. This is a LOT harder to do that it sounds, but the benefits are incredible.

• **Stretch** — Make stretching something you do regularly, especially if you work in an office setting or have a sedentary job. You don't have to spend an hour at it, though. Stretch your body in different directions every few minutes. Stretching enhances muscle and joint flexibility, which prevents you from frequent injuries.

• **Spend Time with Your Loved Ones** — Exercise is all well and good, but exercising with your loved ones is even better. The level of the motivation behind such a routine is unmatched. Working out with your friends and family members also makes the entire routine fun, and you are likely to engage them often.

CHAPTER 4

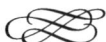

CREATING GOALS FOR SUCCESS

*W*e need to set ourselves up for success, and there are many different areas that we can focus on to achieve this. We started by creating a vision of yourself that we are trying to obtain. That's a great first step, but now we need to get specific. We do this by setting goals, and more specifically, we are setting S.M.A.R.T. goals.

SMART Goals

You have many targets towards achieving your ultimate goal. Some of the goals might be about results and others about the process. Whatever the case, ensure they meet the following conditions:

- **Specific** — Specificity is key to quality goal setting. "I want to exercise" is a very vague goal. However, "I want to run for half an hour every morning" is clearer and more realistic. The more specific, the better, and the more likely you will actually achieve the goal.

- **Measurable** — Ensure your goals can be set against a standard gauge for the purpose of objectivity. This will also help you know whether you are making progress or not. In the example above, running for half an hour every morning is a measurable goal. A half hour is a measure of time. You could also say you would like to run for a measurable distance like 3 miles. Whatever your goal, make sure it is measurable.

• **Attainable** — Think about the time and the other resources available to you when planning your goals. Attainable goals are realistic, and you can work hard to achieve them. Say you want to run in the New York City Marathon, but that is taking place in 3 weeks. That goal is not attainable and therefore wouldn't qualify as a SMART goal. A more attainable goal would be to run in a marathon in 12 months. This would give you more than enough time to prepare.

• **Relevant** — Why is it important for you to achieve the goals you have outlined? Your goals must be about you, and no one else. Don't allow someone else to set your goals. Don't copy their goals either. Your lives and bodies are different, and you are working towards different objectives.

• **Time-Conscious** — Your goals must have a time limit within which you can achieve them. Give yourself a target and work hard to beat it. Say you want to run for half an hour every morning. What distance do you want to cover in that time? This can form the basis for evaluating your progress.

Setting Weight Loss Goals

Did you know that losing even 5% of your total body weight can make a big difference? To get there, you must have specific weight loss goals that will guide your progress. The steps below will help you develop relevant weight loss goals that will not only keep you motivated but will also help you focus.

One of the reasons why we are ditching fad diets is because their focus is on short-term results. Short-term results give you an illusion of progress before your body slumps back into default overweight settings. The frustration that comes with such developments has seen many people develop a negative outlook on their lives and become anxious about social interactions because they are not comfortable with what is happening to them. Planning for the long-term is a different ball game altogether. Think of this like driving a car. When you are driving, you aren't looking at what is directly in front of the car. You are looking much further down the road to see what is ahead. The same principle applies to healthy habits that will eventually lead to weight loss. The core objective here is to live a healthy lifestyle. To do this, you must create simple lifestyle habits that you are happy about, and can help you keep your weight within a manageable level over time. Long-term changes will also involve altering your eating plan and embracing a fitness routine.

Gradual and steady progress is critical to your weight loss goals. The progress you make when you follow this method is steady and will last. Unless you give up before you accomplish your objectives, you won't have to worry about lost weight coming back to haunt you.

Since you have an idea of the ultimate objective, break it down into smaller, manageable milestones. It is essentially impossible to achieve a long-term plan overnight. Smaller goals that are achievable in the short-term are manageable, which makes them easier to work towards. Say you want to lose nine pounds in three months. You can break this down into three pounds every month. By the end of the first month, when you realize you have lost three pounds or more, you will be excited and motivated to continue until you reach your ultimate objectives. You will then build on this success. You had a specific and measurable goal, and you achieved them. Great job, keep up the good work.

Always track your progress. Keep a journal where you

indicate your goals for each week, what you did, and your statistics from the previous week. Today, there are many apps you can use for this to track your progress from your phone. You can also list your goals on a whiteboard in your bedroom where you can see them every day as a reminder of what you are working towards.

Also, don't be afraid to reset your goals as needed. Your goals towards healthy living and weight loss should not be fixed. Embrace flexible goals that you can adjust accordingly. Things change in your life all the time, and this might have an impact on your goals. Instead of giving up when things don't go your way, tweak your plan a bit and get back on the road. Adjustments are especially necessary around vacations, holidays, and special events when you might have to step outside your healthy meal plan.

Weight Tracking

Once you have outlined your weight loss goals, the next step is to find a way to track your progress. Include a reward each time you meet or beat your targets so that you are motivated to work harder next time. One of the ways I did this was by planning a vacation. I knew I wanted to be at a certain weight for a beach trip, so I made it a goal to be at a certain weight by a certain date.

Weight tracking helps you recognize the progress you have made, and how much further you need to go

Why is it important for you to log your progress? The following are some of the reasons why:

• Provides a reinforcing and motivating approach that reminds you why you are working out

• Keeps you grounded and committed to your long-term plans

• Makes it easier to work towards your goals and surpass them

- Helps in accountability for your goals and for yourself
- Uses the tracking report to identify areas where you need to modify your plan
- Helps you plan your time wisely and efficiently

Don't just track your weight loss habits; track the food you eat, too. It is easier to lose weight when you are aware of how much food you are eating and the ingredients. If you feel overwhelmed at some point, discuss your situation with an expert or reevaluate your plans.

Determine Your Macros

It is important that we set the right goals for our weight loss journey. If we have our goal weight and we know our current weight, how do we set up a plan to get there? I would recommend seeing a dietician so they can give you a customized plan that is tailored to your body.

The first step that you can take is to determine your Macros.

What Are Macros?

Of the food we eat, they are comprised of three macronutrients. They are carbohydrates, protein and fat. For example, pasta is high in carbs where chicken is high in protein but low in fat.

You can use a macro calculator to tell you the best ratio of macros that you should eat in order to reach your ideal weight. Knowing this information allows you to monitor and track the food you eat each day to ensure you are on the right path.

I recommend this approach due to its high success rate as well as the fact that it allows you to eat the foods you love!

There are many macro calculators online that will walk you through the steps, where you put in your Age, Gender, Height, Weight, Activity Level, Goal Weight and it will spit out the ideal Calorie Count for each day as well as your ideal ratio of Protein, Fat and Carbs. It can be customized to your goal. If you want to lose weight, it will tell you the macros to achieve that. Once you reach your ideal weight, it will tell you the macros to maintain that weight. Hop on Google and search Macro Calculator and get started!

CHAPTER 5

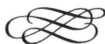

CREATING AN ENVIRONMENT OF
SUCCESS

*A*lot is going on when you step outside your home. It is very important that you are creating an environment of success where you reside. It is important that you do everything you can do to facilitate your transition into a healthy weight loss regime.

The concept here is to answer a simple question: what can you do about your home to make it healthier and more enabling environment for weight loss? Here are some things you can consider:

• **Keep Your Kitchen Clean** — Each time you come to the kitchen and see the mess, you might take the easy way out and order delivery from the nearest restaurant. It is important that your kitchen is inviting and usable. Make sure you have proper utensils to cook and eat at home.

• **Declutter the Fridge** — Get rid of the junk. It is important to get rid of all the excess clutter that accumulates in your fridge over time. If it isn't a healthy ingredient that you plan on using to cook your healthy meals, get rid of it. Out with the old and in with the new.

• **Get Rid of Junk Food**— Have you heard the saying 'abs

are made in the kitchen'? It is true. Even with hours of exercise, all of that effort is wasted if you aren't eating healthy. A healthy diet and proper portion control are the main ingredients to a healthy lifestyle. That is why it is so important for you to stop buying junk food. As long as it is present in your house, it will be difficult for you to resist the urge to eat it. There is enough temptation outside of your home; there is no reason to bring it around you.

• **Never Grocery Shop on An Empty Stomach** — Research has shown that when you shop at the grocery store when you are hungry, you are more likely to purchase high-calorie foods. You know the feeling of being hungry and everything you see looks good. This will cause you to bring back unhealthy foods, which you will eventually eat. Along those same lines, another good rule when grocery shopping is to always bring a list with you. Plan ahead and be intentional with what foods you buy. Stick to the list and you won't be tempted to reach for the junk food. Also, in traditional grocery stores, stick to the outside aisles. This is where most of the healthy foods are located. All the junk foods are in the middle aisles, so try and avoid those if possible.

External Support System

You can't also control outside influences, but you can you do your best to create a positive environment. When people around you are aware of your desire to lose weight, they will try to hold you accountable. They remind you that you are in this together, and the fruits of seeing your fitness and healthy meal regime all the way through will outweigh any feelings of self-doubt you are going through at the moment.

Working out with someone helps keep you motivated. Exercise is more enjoyable when someone else is engaging in it with you. You can also challenge one another to go the extra mile, over and above what you set out to achieve for the day.

Things will not always be easy. There could be setbacks and injuries involved. Having a support system helps because they help you brave these difficult periods in your plan, and give you hope that you will overcome your challenges and get back to your fitness goals in no time.

Keeping appointments is another reason why having a support system is important. When you schedule a training session with a friend, you try your best to make it on time. You don't want to let them down. In essence, you are committing to your plans but your mind tells you that you are doing it, so you don't let your partner or friend down.

Having a workout companion creates a team spirit. You belong to a team of two or more, so you will always work hard for the collective benefit of everyone else.

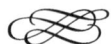

CHAPTER 6

PORTION CONTROL AND MINDFUL EATING HABITS

$\mathcal{F}$ad diets are all the rage today. They are endorsed by celebrities and people who have a huge following online, which makes it easier for most of their followers to get onboard. These diets are not useful. They do not add value to your life. They are only effective in the short-term.

Sustainable weight loss is not about achieving a single short-term goal; it is about losing weight and keeping it off. The celebrities and advocates of the fad diets are people whose desire is to lose weight quickly for a specific reason. Once they achieve their purpose, they get on with their lives without necessarily trying to maintain those initial results.

While there are so many diets out there with different conditions and meal plans, they all seem to agree on one thing: portion control. At least there is one good thing you can learn from them, right?

Portion control supersedes fad diets and any other diet. Portion control is a habitual change that will have a lasting impact on your life (Zuraikat, Roe, Sanchez, & Rolls, 2018). Why do we need portion control? What has brought us to this exact moment where we need to view portion control as the way forward?

We have lost touch with what it means to eat healthily. Everywhere you look, there is a fast food restaurant or some specialty restaurant that offers amazing delicacies. Most of the menus in these restaurants are so carefully crafted, you take one look at them and you feel like you could eat the entire restaurant. Well, that works for the marketing department and the restaurant, but not for you, the one person whose opinion should matter. After all, it is your health that is at stake here.

Another analogy would be the average food portions. A lot has changed over the years. Today, we have dinner plates as large as 13 inches in diameter, while the average plate size a few decades ago used to be no more than 9 inches in diameter (Purdy, 2019). Almost everywhere you go, there is a lot of emphasis on offering more food at a cheaper price. This is what we consider value addition today. It might look like value addition, but to be honest, it is not even close.

In this instance, you are looking at value addition in terms of how much you spend on a plate with a large quantity of food. If you can get more food at a lower price, then you've succeeded. This is the notion that has gone around and become the norm.

The problem with this analogy is that, in your desire to spend less and eat more, you end up creating a cycle where you progressively overeat. Ask anyone today and they can name a few restaurants where you can eat an excessive amount of food at a very low cost. If you think this is not true, see how people get excited at the prospect of an all-you-can-eat buffet.

In short, society has embraced gigantic portions, and somehow, we feel it is okay to keep at it. Wrong! You need to learn how to control your portions (Scott, 2019). This is the only way you will manage to keep your weight in check.

Is Portion Control Effective?

There are a lot of techniques that have been proposed to help you manage your meals and appetite. You can try as many of them as you want, but as long as you are still going after all the food that's in front of you to excess, you are doing it wrong.

Try to eat less food over time. This is a technique that has been suggested so many times. However, it only works well in the short-term. It will only be a matter of time before you get back to your former habits of clearing everything on your plate. Before you know it, you are struggling with obesity (Hook, 2009). So, what can you do about your portions? How do you create a habit that is sustainable, and will help you overcome overeating problems over the long term? Here are some useful ideas that will work for you:

• **Intuitive Portion Control** — You might not always have a scale to determine how much food you need. Instead, learn how to estimate the right portions without using a scale. If you have a scale, measure the right ingredients and transfer them into your hands. This gives you experience in estimating the right quantities if you are ever in a situation where you don't have a scale.

• **Plan Your Meals** — Planning is important for anything you need to succeed in, especially portion control. Think about it this way; before you embraced portion control, you would go out and eat whatever you want, whenever you wanted. These are the things you need to change. There are a lot of things that are wrong with your current eating habits, and you cannot change all of them at once. Come up with a plan. Your plan addresses your present immediate problems and helps you figure out a way to tackle them. Some of the things you need to identify are your hunger triggers, obstacles, and routines that you can initiate to make portion control easier. The good thing about planning is that it sets the tone for evaluation. With a plan, you can review your meal habits after a while and determine whether you have made any progress or not. This will also guide you as you fully embrace portion control.

• **Get Some Portion Control Plates** — After planning, the next step is to ensure you have all the tools and equipment ready. Portion control plates are useful here. Buy smaller plates if you have to. With each meal, try to include more fruits and vegetables.

• **Embrace the 2-in-1 Meal Plan** — Assuming you eat out at one of the restaurants where meals are served in large portions, you do not have to finish all the food at once. Ask the restaurant to pack the rest of your food to-go. You don't have to do this after you have eaten. Instead, ask before you start eating, so they can pack half of your food for later use.

• **Keep the Leftovers** — Do not throw away the leftovers when you prepare meals at home. Keep them for later consumption. Unpacking leftovers for your next meal might help you eat less. In your mind, you are aware that you have some food remaining from the previous meal. Therefore, you do not have to prepare more food. Leftovers also help you stop eating out of the house for convenience.

• **Introduce Vegetables** — We will discuss vegetables at length in the next chapter, including their benefits and why you should add more of them to your diet. Vegetables are low-calorie foods. This is one of the reasons why you need to include them in your diet. They are full of antioxidants, vitamins, and minerals (Gottlieb, 2003). Their low-calorie rating makes them a better alternative to many other foods that might be on your list. While vegetables are a healthy addition to your meals, not everyone loves them. If you had a difficult time eating vegetables when you were younger, chances are high that you might have kept up the habit into your adult life. An easier way to overcome this is to introduce vegetables into your diet gradually. Add vegetables on the side with every meal. This is something simple, but it will go a long way in helping you with your weight decisions. You can create a list of a variety of vegetables you can throw into your meals from time to time. The best thing about vegetables is that they complement virtually every meal.

• **Choose Your Cooking Oil Wisely** — Which oil do you use to cook? Think about using healthier alternatives like olive oil, safflower oil, or canola oil rather than butter, shortening, or coconut oil, which have a lot of saturated fat. Remember that all your meals do not necessarily need oil. You can steam some foods to keep them fresh and nutritious and still enjoy them.

• **Prepare Portion-Controlled Meals** — It is nearly impossible for you to adhere to portion control when you are hungry and tired after a difficult day at work. When this happens, you might end up eating too much food. If you prepare portion-controlled meals ahead of time, you can reach into your refrigerator, pick what you need, and eat it without worrying about going overboard.

• **Prepare Food for One** — Are you the type of person who prepares all their food on Sunday for the week ahead? This is a good idea to keep your week organized, especially if you are prone to having busy work weeks. If you do this, do not store the food in bulk. Instead, prepare single-serving packages and put the food away like that. This makes your work easier during the week because all you have to do is pick one serving, warm the food, and be on your way.

• **Learn Portion Control** — It is not easy to start something abruptly. The same applies to portion control. When you are ready, allow yourself a window period where you learn how to do it. This is more of an experimenting phase.

Portion control is not something you will start and get right immediately, especially if you have been overeating. If you attempt this, you might feel disillusioned and fall back into your former habits sooner than you think. The best way to go about this is to introduce changes gradually and notice the effect over a few weeks. You can give yourself at least a month to see how your body is adjusting to the new changes.

• **Manage Your Serving Sizes** — Portion control is about knowing the ideal portion size for you. While earlier on you were eating uncontrollably, when you embrace portion control, you have a limit beyond which you know you are overeating. It makes it worse that food portions are larger in many restaurants today, and, for this reason, a lot of people struggle to figure out their ideal portion. One tactic that will help you here is to read food labels. Food labels contain all the nutritional information about the food you buy. This is easier if you are buying food to prepare meals at home. You need to read these labels, or you will fall into a marketing trap. Remember that, while manufacturers try to offer you healthy eating options, their ultimate goal is profit margins. The person who cares the most about your eating habits is you. But what about if you are eating at a friends house or are at a restaurant? It can be tricky to know how much food to put on your plate. There is a simple solution by using your hands and fists as a reference. Your fist, palms, and thumbs can tell you what one portion of rice, meat, or fat looks like. A clenched fist equals about one cup. The front of your closed fist equals about half a cup. Your fingertip is about one teaspoon. Your entire thumb is equal to about one tablespoon. Your palm is equal to about one portion of meat or fish.

Let's break it down even more for everyday use.
• Your palm determines your protein portions.
• Your fist determines your veggie portions.

- Your cupped hand determines your carb portions.
- Your thumb determines your fat portions.

Protein:

To determine your protein intake, here are some suggested serving sizes. As with everything else, consult a dietician for their suggested amount.

For protein-dense foods like meat, fish, eggs, dairy, or beans, use a palm-sized serving. For men, we recommend two palm-sized portions with each meal. And for women, one palm-sized portion with each meal is what is recommended.

Veggies:

For veggies like broccoli, spinach, etc.– use a cupped hand to determine your serving size. For men, we recommend 2 cupped-hand sized portions of carbohydrates with most meals. For women, one cupped hand.

Carbs:

For carbohydrate-dense foods – like grains, starches, a closed fist is a great reference. One fist of carbs is great when starting out to keep the carbohydrate intake lower, which will accelerate weight loss. Feel free to increase you get closer to your ideal weight.

Learn to Read Food Labels

Many times, we buy food without looking at the nutrition charts. Almost all packaged foods have nutrition charts attached to help you understand the nutrient components of what you are buying (Soederberg Miller, 2016). This is a good way to stay healthy and keep an eye on your meals. Unfortunately, most people do not read food labels. It is common to ignore the labels when you are already aware of what you get from a specific product you are familiar with. However, companies change their production process from time to time, so it is wise to check every time.

Before you look at the nutrition label, there are some

important facts that you must keep at the back of your mind. First, the information displayed on the labels is estimated on a 2000-calorie a day diet. Depending on your physiological needs, you might need more or less. Second, some nutrition labels might indicate 0 grams of trans fat, but you still find partially hydrogenated oil in the list of ingredients. What this means is that the package has some trans-fat, but in each serving, it is less than 0.5 grams. Therefore, if you have more than a single serving, you might be eating more trans-fat. Third, the nutrition label is regulated by the US Food and Drug Administration (FDA). The FDA tries to make it easier for you to identify the amount of added sugars and calories in the product you are purchasing. They also recommend realistic serving sizes.

So, what should you look for in the food labels? There are five important bits of information that you should understand:

1. **Serving Size** — This is the first thing on the nutrition facts table. It indicates what the size of one serving should be, and the estimated number of servings you can expect from the package or container you are buying.

2. **Calories** — From the serving, look at the calories. How many calories are you consuming with each serving? If you ate the entire package, how many calories do you consume? This is simple math. Multiply the number of calories per serving by the number of estimated servings in the package. Is this within your desired range?

3. **Nutrients to Consume in Moderation** — After calories, the next section should reveal the nutrients present in the package you are buying. Read this carefully because some nutrients should be taken in moderation. Take fats, for example. Some fats are good. The composition of sugar might include added and natural sugar. Choose foods that do not contain a lot of added sugars, sodium, or saturated fat.

Speaking of fats, avoid trans-fat as much as possible. This information should act as a guideline for you whenever you are trying to compare and choose between different food labels.

4. **Important Nutrients** — In the next section, the manufacturer indicates all the important vitamins and minerals present in the package you are buying. This is where you find things like potassium, magnesium, dietary fiber, calcium, choline, and so forth.

5. **Percentage Daily Value** — Percentage daily value, often indicated as %DV, shows you how many nutrients are available in each ideal daily serving. This should guide you, especially if you plan on preparing meals that contain a specific percentage of a given nutrient.

Mindful Eating

Mindful eating is something very few people talk about, but it will help you stay healthy and manage your eating habits properly. Instead of going on a diet that will do more harm than good, being mindful of what you eat can make a big difference in your life. Mindful eating can help you stop binge eating and will help you feel better about yourself and your health.

Through mindful eating, you learn how to pay attention to your experiences in real life. This depends on physical cues and listening to your cravings. We often run to food when we think we are hungry, but in a real sense, we are not. We are just glorifying a craving for something else, or we are projecting our stress onto our meals.

Mindful eating is a wholesome process that will include the following changes in the way you approach your meals:

• **Appreciate the Food You Eat** — This is something we don't often do. We just eat because we can, without thinking about why we need the food we eat.

- Identify the Connection Between Your Body, Feelings, and Food
- Eat Food with the Purpose of Maintaining a Healthy Lifestyle
- **Manage and Cope with the Pressure** — You may deal with pressures concerning food, anxiety, and guilt, especially if you were, or still are, an overeater.
- **Use Your Senses** — Embrace your meals with all your senses, including sound, taste, texture, smell, and color. This helps you enjoy the food you eat.
- Identify How Real Hunger Feels
- Learn How to Eat Slowly Without Being Distracted

Mindfulness is a technique that has helped many people seeking cognitive therapy become more aware about their health, and responses (Galante, Iribarren, & Pearce, 2012). A lot of the mental disorders that people overcome through mindfulness are usually the result of distorted automatic thoughts that they have held in their subconscious for quite some time.

If you can change the way you think about food and your behavior towards it, you can learn to embrace a new, better approach to eating, and in the long run, lose weight without going through an arduous and irrelevant diet to achieve your desired weight. Through mindfulness, you will embrace new techniques that you can introduce into your life gradually, which will become your new way of life. This is probably the most effortless way to lose weight without the risk of gaining the weight back.

Why Should You Consider Mindful Eating?

Think about the society we live in. There is barely enough time for you to do everything to get through the day. People are multitasking everywhere to get so many things done in a short amount of time. Our jobs are so demanding that we are losing the connection we have with society and, more importantly, our families, loved ones, and ourselves. One of the important things that have suffered in the process is the way we eat.

If you visit any busy workplace, mealtimes are no longer the mealtimes we were used to when growing up. Most people eat while working or doing something else. More focus is placed on their other tasks, instead of their food. This fast-paced life has also seen a shift from healthy food towards fast food options, which keep springing up at the corners of every new office block. It is almost impossible to walk a few blocks without bumping into a fast food chain.

Other than the unhealthy food choices, there are many distractions you will come across, which divert your attention from food. The most notorious are smartphones, computers, TV, social media, and gaming. It is amazing how someone can start eating while engaging in any of the above, but barely five minutes in, they put their food aside to focus on the distraction. By the time you get back to your food, it is cold and you might not even have an appetite anymore.

As a result, eating has moved from one of the most important things in our day to just another activity that we need to rush through. Did you know that the brain needs roughly twenty minutes to decode signals from your hormones that you are full? Therefore, if you are rushing through your meals in five minutes or less, you can do so much damage before your brain realizes you exceeded your limit. This is one of the challenges of binge eating.

Mindfulness empowers you to realize your body's cues when you are hungry or full, so you can act accordingly (Masuda & Hill, 2013). There is a big difference between emotional hunger and physical hunger. Both of these need unique attention. When you are aware of the trigger, you can isolate it from your responses, allowing you sufficient time to determine the best approach for every situation.

How Mindfulness Supports Weight Loss

By now, you are well aware of the fact that all those weight loss diets will not work in the long run. In fact, you might end up even worse off than when you started. Lack of awareness of your eating patterns is one of the reasons why binge eating spirals out of control. Even if you lose weight, responding to all your cravings through comfort food will result in you gaining weight again, which can be very frustrating and discouraging.

Mindfulness allows you to embrace your life, reflect on what you do, and determine how to address your poor behavior towards food (Schultz, 2017). When you do this, you have a better shot at long-term success with weight loss. You will not be addressing weight loss from the symptoms; instead, you will address weight loss from the perspective of the things that make you gain weight in the first place. You do away with your unhealthy habits.

Mindful Eating Guidelines

You need to be more aware of your eating habits, but that is easier said than done. How do you go about it? What should you do? Remember that it is the simple changes you make that will go a long way in helping you overcome your obstructive patterns. Here is a simple checklist of what to do:

- **Eat Slowly** — Do not be in a hurry to wolf down your food. This is one of the reasons why some people end up choking on their food. Sit down and eat without rushing, allowing your body to digest the food comfortably.

- **Chew Your Food** — Many people bite into their food and swallow it almost immediately. You cannot fully enjoy your food if you eat this way. Depending on the food you are eating, you need to chew at least twenty times before you swallow it. The longer the food stays in your mouth, the more time it allows your taste buds to identify the flavors, and you will love the food even more. While at it, remember to eat in small bites. You can taste all the flavors when your mouth is not completely full. In fact, it is advisable that you put your utensils down after each bite so you can savor the taste. Between the moment you bite the food and the time you swallow, involve all your senses. This is not something a lot of people think about, but it helps. Recognize the aroma, the color, the ingredients, seasonings, and so forth. These are the things that will help you enjoy what you eat and look forward to another meal.

- **Appreciate the Food You Eat** — Before you start eating, take a moment to appreciate the food before you. Think about the people who prepared the food, the preparation process, and everything else that was necessary to get the food to your table. This is also the time you will realize that you have some amazing company each time you are eating, which is a valuable experience many people do not get to experience – sharing hearty meals with people who are dear to you.

- **Put your fork down after each bite** - It takes roughly 20 minutes for your stomach to send the message to your brain that you have had enough food. In part, this is one of the reasons why fast food is so unhealthy. It's not just that it's full of empty calories; it's that you can eat it faster than it takes your body to realize you are full. To avoid this, you need to remember to pace yourself through your meal. Put your fork down after each bite, chew thoroughly, and even stop to chat with a friend. You'll find that you'll begin to feel full as you eat more slowly instead of feeling like you're about to pop when you finish all of your food.

- **Eat Reasonable Portions** — Try to limit the size of your plate. On average, your plate should not be more than nine inches in diameter. A larger plate encourages you to fill it up with food. Once it is full, you are under more pressure to eat all the food on the plate. This is a mental trick that causes you to overeat without you realizing it. If you use smaller plates, you train your mind to recognize that you have eaten enough when you clear your plate. Most Americans eat two to three times the actual serving size of foods.

• To make matters worse, restaurants often serve massive portions, which can train your mind to think that's the amount of food your body needs. If you look at the same amount of food on a little plate vs. a large one, your eyes might convince you there's more delicious food on the smaller dish. This is due to what's known as the Delboeuf illusion, which shows that surrounding something in a lot of white space can make it look smaller. Even if you're not eating much, cutting back on the amount of plate space around your food can trick your brain into thinking it's a bigger portion than it really is, whereas doing the opposite may stoke your hunger by making you think you only ate a bit.

• **Don't multitask while you are eating** - It can be tough to focus on eating when there's work to do and social media to check. Eating your meals when you're distracted can lead to accidentally taking in more than you need. Distracted eating doesn't just lead to more consumption at the moment, it can even compel you to eat more than necessary later on in the day.

• **Keep Gum Handy** - This might by my favorite habit that I started doing that had the biggest impact. If you find yourself with a larger portion on your plate than you should be eating, or you find yourself getting full before you are done with the food on your plate, pop in a piece of gum.

• **Respect Your Appetite** — Do you ever pay attention to your appetite? People who skip meals, as is advocated in so many diets, turn up for their meals when they are famished. At this point, you are not looking forward to the meal because you have a healthy appetite, but because you are ravenous and need to get something inside your stomach. Your priority is not to enjoy your meal, but to fill that emptiness. The fastest way to overeat is when your brain is in starvation mode and you want to take in as much food as possible. It is ok to eat healthy snacks in between meals to help reduce those hunger pains.

- **Be a smart snacker** - When you're trying to lose weight, snacking can either be your best friend or your worst enemy. It's important to remember that you need to stay within your predetermined macros for the day in order to be in a caloric deficit. If you snack the right way with healthy veggies that aren't calorie dense, it is a great way to curb your hunger pains until your next meal If you eat unhealthy snacks throughout the day, those calories can quickly add up, even if you are sticking to a healthy diet during your normal meals. Another snacking problem can arise if you graze, aka eat mindlessly throughout the day, rather than snack intentionally.

- **Check Your Shopping List** — Everything starts with your shopping list. We put it last intentionally so you can go through the meal ordeal and understand what you are trying to overcome first, before you go shopping. Shopping calls for planning. Since you are now aware of what your meal times are about, go back to the drawing board and rethink your normal shopping list. Each item you include on this list should have some nutritional value. Avoid foods that do not add value to your meals. While shopping, follow your list carefully so that you do not engage in impulse purchases. Impulse purchases are often things you do not need and can do without, like junk food and processed foods. Try to fill your list with foods in the fresh produce section as much as possible. Read the food labels, so you know how much nutritional value you are getting from your meals. Once you embrace mindful eating, it will become an effortless process and something you do without giving it much thought. Guaranteed, it will not be easy at first, but you are committed to making simple, small changes that will have a lasting impact on your life.

Importance of Vegetables in Your Meal Plan

From your childhood years, your parents and caregivers were always adamant that you need to eat your vegetables. There is a good reason for this. All those years of eating broccoli were not in vain. Even if you complained about it, your mom knew best!

The American Cancer Society advises that you need at least five vegetable and fruit servings daily to maintain a healthy life (Lawrence, 1993). Are you having that already? If not, it is not too late to get it right. The beauty of vegetables is that you have quite the variety to choose from, which also means budgetary restrictions should not hold you back. There is always something you can buy to switch things up so that your vegetable choices do not become boring. Vegetables should be an important part of your meals for the following reasons:

• **Fighting Cancer** — Everyone is worried about cancer right now, and for a good reason. The cost of cancer treatments is insane for an illness that has no definite cure. One of the most important reasons why you need to eat more vegetables is because of this. Unfortunately, many people are succumbing to different cancers every day. Vegetables can lower your risk of getting cancer because of their vitamin C content. Vitamin C helps your body fight illnesses and reduce your exposure to them. Some of the vegetables you can consider include broccoli, parsley, Brussels sprouts, and red bell pepper.

• **Radiant Skin** — Vegetables also help in promoting healthy, radiant skin. Carrots, bell peppers, and tomatoes have a high concentration of carotenoids. These are very powerful antioxidants in the form of beta carotene and vitamin A. Carotenoids are the compounds responsible for the fresh and bright color that vegetables have.

• **Weight Loss** — Most vegetables contain close to zero sugars or saturated fats. The low-fat content makes them ideal for weight loss. Apart from that, the fiber and energy density in most vegetables also helps in keeping your weight in check.

• **Fiber** — Vegetables deliver the recommended amount of dietary fiber. You can only get this from plant foods. Fiber helps to remove cholesterol from the arteries, reducing your risk of developing heart disease in the process. It is also because of fiber that your digestive system operates optimally, keeping your blood sugar levels in check, and subsequently reducing your risk of cancer.

• **Antioxidants and Vitamins** — Vegetables have a very high nutritional value. They carry minerals and vitamins that are responsible for maintaining a healthy body. Many vegetables have a high potassium content, which is necessary for a healthy heart and blood pressure.

• **Proper Eyesight** — Carrots have always been recommended to improve your eyesight, especially for children. The same properties are associated with collards, spinach, beet greens, and kale. A diet that is rich in leafy greens will help to protect your eyes.

Importance of Proteins in Your Meal Plan

You need proteins to live a healthy life. Proteins contain amino acids which merge into long chains that perform different roles in the body. Proteins are important for your health because most of their activity is at a cellular level, the basic foundation of your being. Proteins are important for many reasons. While there is a lot of controversy around the health impact of carbs and fat, there is almost a unanimous consensus across the divide when it comes to proteins. Here are some reasons why you need to eat more proteins:

• **Managing Hunger and Appetite** — One of the challenges that many people face when dealing with weight issues is managing their appetite and hunger. Protein is a fulfilling macronutrient. It makes you feel satisfied faster, without eating too much. Proteins achieve this by reducing the production of ghrelin, the hunger hormone, while encouraging the body to produce more of the YY peptide, the hormone responsible for satiety (Feinle-Bisset, Patterson, Ghatei, Bloom, & Horowitz, 2005). If you are serious about weight loss, or if you need to get rid of accumulated belly fat, replace some of the fats and carbs in your meal plan with proteins. Subtle changes, like reducing the size of your rice serving and adding some slices of fish or meat will go a long way.

• **Increased Strength and Muscle Mass** — Protein is the foundation of your muscles. You need to eat more protein, so you remain stronger. As the building block, you also need proteins to help your body generate your muscles faster, especially if you engage in some form of strength training or contact sport. People who are very active must grow their lean muscle. This particularly holds for athletes. Protein in your diet will also help prevent the risk of muscle loss when you lose weight.

• **Necessary for Healthy Bones** — Individuals who eat more protein have better bone mass as they grow older. This also means they have a lower risk of fractures or osteoporosis. For women, this is an important factor you should not ignore because, after menopause, you have a higher risk of developing osteoporosis. In addition to eating protein, try to embrace an active lifestyle.

• **Supports Healthy Fat Burning and Metabolism** — Your body's metabolism improves when you are eating. This happens because the body burns calories to absorb the nutrients in the food you eat. This is known as the thermic effect of food. Different foods have varying thermic effects. Proteins have a higher thermic effect than carbs or fat. Increasing your protein intake increases your metabolism, and, as a result, the number of calories your body burns.

• **Managing Cravings** — We have discussed this earlier – the difference between food cravings and normal hunger. Cravings are often about the brain demanding some form of reward. While it can be difficult to control cravings, it is not impossible. You can start by preventing them from happening in the first place. Increasing your protein intake is one of the best ways of going about this. Proteins make you feel full, so you do not feel the need to have a snack at night. Late-night snacks are often unhealthy, and most of those snack choices do not have any nutritional value.

• **Reduce Blood Pressure** — Kidney disease, strokes, and heart attacks are all linked to high blood pressure. High protein intake is one of the simplest ways of lowering your blood pressure. Proteins reduce your blood pressure and the level of triglycerides and LDL cholesterol in the blood.

• **Maintain Weight Loss Progress** — It is one thing to lose weight, but it is more difficult to keep that weight off. High protein intake increases your body's metabolic rate. Therefore, your body burns more calories and your desire to indulge in cravings also reduces significantly. These are healthy ways of losing and keeping the weight away.

• **Stay Fit as You Grow Older** — Your muscles and bones weaken as you grow older. This is an obstacle we all experience at some point. However, you do not necessarily have to be very weak just because you are old. You have probably seen many older people who are still strong in their later years. Bone fractures, frailty, and low quality of life in older adults are associated with sarcopenia. Eating more protein can help you reduce the level of deterioration as you grow older, and even keep you from developing sarcopenia. You must also embrace an active lifestyle, like resistance training and lifting weights, to support this.

Benefits of Carbonated Water

Carbonated water is water with carbon dioxide dissolved in it under pressure. This is what gives it the effervescence that is similar to other carbonated drinks like soda. However, there is more to carbonated water than fizz. It is a healthy addition to your meal plan.

Carbonated water has many benefits in your meal plan. It allows your stomach to settle by inducing flatulence or burping, which helps you avoid reflux disease symptoms and reduce pressure in the gut.

Compared with most drinks, carbonated water gives you the illusion of satiety. You avoid having to indulge in food unnecessarily to satisfy your cravings. While carbonated water offers these benefits, when you drink a lot of if you might feel bloated. This is due to the effect of carbon dioxide in the water.

Healthy Meal Habits for a Healthy Life

The following are some tips that are helpful to follow in order to maximize the benefits you can get during your meals:

• **Enjoy Your Company** — There is nothing better than enjoying your meals in the right company. You create stronger and more satisfying bonds, and the conversations are amazing. You frequently look forward to sharing your meals with company. Because of the conversations taking place, you also have a tendency to eat more slowly than when you are eating alone.

• **Eat Lots of Vegetables and Fruits** — Add a lot of vegetables and fruits to your diet. Everyone knows how important these ingredients are, but very few people follow this rule. When possible, fill up at least half of your plate with vegetables and fruits. This is a neat trick that helps you eat healthy food without consuming an overabundance of calories. Instead of reaching for an unhealthy dessert, enjoy a fruit cup instead. Your body will recognize the sweet flavors and will satisfy those sweet tooth cravings you might have after a meal.

• **Introduce More Variety to Your Meals** — Eating the same meals all the time can be boring. After a while, you lose enthusiasm for your meals and easily pick up unhealthy food habits, like eating out all the time. Add some variety to your meal plan, which will keep your food exciting. Find out which healthy meals work for you and start to play around with variations. If you do not like to cook, then find a way to prepare healthy meals in the shortest amount of time possible. Alternatively, if you look to cook, then find different variations of those ingredients that you would like to explore. Take ownership of what you are putting into your body but make it work on your own terms.

• **Recognize Your Hunger Signals** — Everyone has a limit on the amount of food they can eat every day. This depends on different physiological factors like age, gender, weight, and base activity level. Your eating limit will, therefore, not be the same as everyone else's. Listen to your body, so you know when to stop eating, even if you have not cleared your plate. Besides, it is not mandatory that you clear your plate.

• **Hydrate** — Water plays an important role in your health. It helps you avoid fatigue and headaches, and it can help you think clearly. Ensure you have a reusable water bottle wherever you go. Water is your body's principal chemical component and makes up about 60 percent of your body weight. Your body depends on water to survive. Every cell, tissue and organ in your body needs water to work properly.

So how much water does the average, healthy adult need? The National Academies of Sciences, Engineering, and Medicine determined that an adequate daily fluid intake is:
- About 15.5 cups (3.7 liters) of fluids for men
- About 11.5 cups (2.7 liters) of fluids a day for women
- **Respect Your Meal Times** — Do not skip meals. Space your meals accordingly to allow your body enough time to digest and metabolize the food. Apart from the meal times, ensure you eat a healthy and fulfilling breakfast, followed by an average-sized lunch and a light dinner. This helps you sleep well at night and wake up feeling energetic.

Useful Weight Loss Tips

Having considered the discussion points above, the following are some simple, quick tips that you can keep at the back of your mind. You can implement them in your life gradually as you lose weight and keep it off for good:
- **Get Enough Sleep** — One of the reasons many people gain weight is poor sleeping patterns. Make sure you are getting quality sleep every day. If you are not, reevaluate your sleeping arrangements. Poor sleep has repeatedly been linked to weight gain. Everyone's sleep requirements vary, but it is important to get at least 8 hours of sleep at night. Poor sleep can also decrease your metabolism.
- **Track Your Weight** — Try to check your weight often. This will help you stay on track and see how you are progressing towards your goals. I purchased a digital scale that would link to an app (MyFitnessPal). This made it easy for me to see what my current weight is, how much progress I have made and how much further I need to go to reach my goal weight.
- **Eat More Unprocessed, Whole Foods** — Unprocessed, whole foods should feature in your diet more often. These foods are not just healthier, they are also more fulfilling and you will have a lower chance of overeating.

• **Eat Slowly** — This goes back to mindful eating. People who eat too quickly have a higher risk of adding weight. Eating slowly allows you to control the amount of food you consume, and you can stop when you feel full.

• **Enjoy Your Tea and Coffee** — Tea and coffee boost your body's metabolism. When you first start losing weight, it is common to feel a little sluggish. Tea and Coffee (without the unhealthy sugars and creamers) are a great pick-me-up to keep you motivated until your next meal or workout. As long as you do it in moderation.

• **Eat More Soluble Fiber** — Soluble fibers can help to reduce the amount of fat accumulated in your belly area.

• **Buy Foods That Support Your Weight Loss Goals** — Be mindful about your shopping list. Make sure you buy foods that will help you achieve your weight loss objectives (Gunnars, 2018).

• **Hydrate Before Your Meals** — Drink water at least half an hour before your meal time. This will help in digestion.

• **Avoid Fruit Juice and Sugary Drinks** — Fruit juice and sugary drinks contribute to weight gain. If you can stay away from them, you have a better chance of living a healthy, lean life.

• **High-Protein Breakfast** — This is your first meal of the day. A high-protein meal will reduce your cravings and help you avoid unnecessary calorie consumption during the day. Starting your day right is the best way to stay on course with your weight loss goals.

• **It is recommended that you eat your food sitting down at a table, and from a small plate**. The reason for this is that food eaten out of packages and while standing is quickly consumed. The unintentional result is that you wind up eating much more than if you sat down and consciously enjoyed your meals.

• **Also, be sure to serve food onto individual plates, and**

leave the extras back where they were prepared. Large portions of food sitting on the table in front of you are tempting you to eat them. It takes incredible will power not to dig in for seconds. Don't forget, it takes about 20 minutes for your mind to get the signal from your belly that you are full.

CHAPTER 7

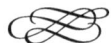

HOW TO SURVIVE IN THE REAL WORLD

So you have eliminated all the junk food from your kitchen, cleaned out your fridge, and no longer go grocery shopping on an empty stomach. That is great! But what about the weekends or when you want to enjoy a night out with friends and family? From time to time, you will want to eat at a restaurant. Perhaps it is a celebration of some sort, or a romantic evening. For someone who has made the bold decision to prepare and enjoy their meals at home, restaurant dining might present certain challenges. If you don't know how to get around them, you could undo the progress you have made in maintaining a healthy weight and start a downward spiral.

Understanding Restaurant Psychology

You might think that the restaurant menu is a collection of dishes randomly organized according to their prices or categories. This is not true. Restaurant owners invest a lot in their menu designs to keep you hooked. Today, we have menu consultants and engineers whose job is to deliver a compelling menu that is easy to read, and highly profitable for the restaurant. You didn't know that until now, did you?

The average restaurant menu is a set of mind tricks that you should not fall for. This is one of the reasons why eating at a restaurant when you are watching your weight is not very easy. When you know what to expect from a restaurant menu, it is easier to walk in with an open mind.

Five-Point Guidelines for Healthy Restaurant Meals

Knowing that you are going to eat out, how do you prepare? Remember that your goal is to keep your calories and portions in check. The following is a five-point plan that will help you stay on track with your weight loss plans without compromising a good night out:

1. **Review the Menu in Advance** — Before you eat at a restaurant, look up their menu options. It is easier to make an informed decision about your food in advance than in the heat of the moment when you might be distracted by good conversation. You might go to a restaurant with a group of friends and start discussing how amazing the food is. Before you know it, your decision is swayed by popular opinion. Many customers do this today, and in response, restaurants are increasingly adding their menus on their websites and social media pages, so that their customers know beforehand what they want to eat. This also makes their work easier, because you can call in advance and reserve a table, and have your meal prepared shortly before you arrive.

2. **Request More Information from the Chef** — Before you place an order, ask if you can speak to the chef for clarification. Ask them about the portion sizes, ingredients, cooking methods, and so on. Many restaurants will allow this. However, you must be polite about your request. If you appear overbearing or rude, they might throw you out altogether. It is okay to ask the chef to modify some ingredients to meet your caloric needs. You are better off asking for this instead of waiting to get surprised. Some meals might get to your table as a larger portion size than you imagined. In such

a case, ask your dining partner to share the meal with you, if possible.

3. **Utilize Appetizers instead of Entrées** — Appetizers can help you with portion control. This is a better alternative than the entrée menu. Appetizers, especially when accompanied by a vegetable side dish or salad, can nourish you without causing you to consume unnecessary calories in the process. Your budget will not suffer a significant dent either!

4. **Avoid Alcohol** — When you are eating in a restaurant, avoid alcohol, or limit yourself to healthier options. Certain alcohols, like beer, are high in carbohydrates, and cocktails often have a very high sugar content and provide no nutritional value. Besides, consuming alcohol impairs your decision-making, increasing your chances of making poor food choices.

5. **Meals-To-Go** — Most restaurant meals come in oversized portions. Instead of soldiering through the meal, ask to split some of the food in a to-go pack before you start eating. This is a brilliant way to make sure you do not eat more calories than you need. Besides, you will not be forcing food mindlessly down your throat when you are already full just because you don't want to waste your money. Dining away from home is not supposed to be the self-sabotaging exercise it has become in recent times. What we have learned here is that you can enjoy your occasional restaurant meal without interfering with your weight loss objectives.

Hacking the Eating out Experience

We are social beings. You will end up going out to eat at some point. It is always fun to catch up with your friends and family members over a meal. This strengthens your bond, and in the process, you can also meet some amazing people. Beyond the social aspect, eating out is one of the reasons why many people over-eat. The risk of overindulgence is very high and combined with alcohol and peer pressure, you make some of the worst food choices when you go out to eat.

For someone who is watching their weight, you do not want to withdraw from your social connections and miss out on the opportunity to have fun with those around you. The following are some useful hacks that will help you enjoy a good time eating out without giving up on your social life or regressing on your weight loss milestones:

Create a list of your most frequented restaurants and decide what you can eat there:

You know the restaurants you frequent the most. Most restaurants will have their menus listed online. Take the time to list out the restaurants you frequent the most and compile a list of meals that you decide are healthy options that you can order next time you visit. Rather than leaving things up to chance and being presented with a full menu of unhealthy options, eliminate the chance for failure and make a list ahead of time. Keep them in your smartphone, so it is easy for you to access before you go to the restaurant. Have a plan in place for when you get there. It is important to stay disciplined when you get there and not be tempted by the other food that is being paraded around to the other patrons. You should feel proud that you are making smart and healthy decisions.

Order first at restaurants:

If it is a restaurant you frequent often, you should already know what you want because you researched ahead of time. If it is a new restaurant, it's even more important to be the first to order so you aren't tempted to get something less healthy because a friend ordered it before you. A University of Illinois study found that people will tend to order similarly when in a group. People are happier making similar choices as their peers. If you tend to be indecisive and rely on hearing what other people are getting, check out the menu at home, decide on a dish, and ask the waiter if you can order first.

Ask for dressing and sauces on the side:

If you let the restaurant dress your salad for you, there is a high chance you will get way too much dressing that suffocates your once-nutritious vegetables. Depending on your dressing of choice, that can set you back anywhere from 300 to 400 calories. Instead, be sure to ask for the dressing on the side and only use half of it to save more than 150 calories.

Grab a Healthy Snack Before:

A healthy snack before you go to the restaurant helps you feel less hungry. By the time you arrive, you will not eat as much as someone who has not eaten anything yet. Consider something like yogurt, which is a low-calorie, high-protein snack. With a half-full stomach, your risk of overeating decreases substantially.

Hydrate:

Drink water before and with your meal. While at it, try to avoid sweetened drinks. Drinking water helps to reduce your consumption of added sugar and unnecessary calories. For extra flavor, add a lemon.

Avoid All-You-Can-Eat Buffets:

These buffets are the last place you want to be if you are eating healthy. In a society where food portions are already larger than life, someone who offers you such a buffet is setting you up for failure. Staying within your limits is very difficult if you are in a place with an unlimited food supply. It gets worse when you are accompanied by your friends or family members. If you cannot get out of a buffet, choose a smaller plate, or ask for one. This will help you control what you eat. In case that is not possible, fill half of your normal-sized plate with vegetables or salad.

Swap Fries for Vegetables:

Most menus offer the main course with a side of french

fries. Rather than eating those extra calories, ask your waiter if they can swap some of your meal with extra salad or vegetables. Most of the time, they will do this at no extra charge. This is a brilliant way to slash your calorie intake while consuming more vegetables.

Avoid the Bread Basket:

Many restaurants offer a pre-dinner bread or chip basket. If you arrive when you are hungry, this is a distraction that gets you into overeating mode before your meal even arrives. If you cannot resist the temptation, ask the waiter to remove the bread basket from the table.

Salad or Soup Starters:

Having a salad or soup before the main course fills you up enough that, by the time your meal arrives, you are not compelled to eat as much. Request vegetable-based sauces instead of cheese- or cream-based sauces to eat healthy and reduce fat and calories from your meal.

Healthy Shopping Guide

Proper nutrition is not just about what you eat; it is also about the ingredients you buy. When you go to the grocery store, you encounter a wide variety of food items that can end up on your plate. Without the right ingredients, you will not make progress towards achieving your weight loss goals.

Grocery shopping is not one of the easiest things to do, especially if you have very specific grocery needs. The choices are numerous and overwhelming, and you must also learn to read the labels to determine what is good for you (American Heart Association, 2018). Coupled with the fact that markets try to manipulate you to buy things you do not need; it is quite a jungle out there. Healthy shopping is not a mirage, however. It is something you can get through without a hitch. It calls for planning, a bit of information, and asking for help where necessary. Attendants are present at the grocery store so that you do not struggle to find what you need.

First, always make sure you have a list before you go shopping. This list helps you stick to the plan. If you are preparing meals for the whole week, your shopping list should account for this. The few minutes you spend making this list will prevent you from running back and forth because you forgot something important. There is no shame in using coupons. In fact, look for some coupons in grocery ads. When you get to the store, factor in the discounts and sales offers when planning your meals. Never go shopping when you are hungry. This increases your risk of impulse buys, and you might end up with ingredients or snacks that are unneeded or unhealthy for your weight plan.

A lot of people find comfort in buying the same foods over and over again. While this is convenient, think about adding some variety in your choices. Do not switch things up drastically. If you opt for variety, introduce it gradually so that you do not upset your meal balance. With these ideas in mind, let's take a look at different food sections at the grocery store and how to navigate them:

• **Fresh Produce** — For a healthy meal plan, this is the section that deserves most of your attention. Different vegetables and fruits have different minerals, vitamins, and phytonutrients. Try to pick your selections from different colors. For your root vegetables, for example, you can buy sweet potatoes and carrots, cabbages and broccoli for your cruciferous vegetables, and kale and lettuce for your leafy greens. For the best flavor, always pick produce that is in season.

• **Pasta, Cereals, and Bread** — Always go for 100% whole grain. If you choose processed ingredients, choose the least processed of them all. Instead of instant oatmeal, for example, choose regular oatmeal. Though whole grain instant oatmeal is still acceptable. To prevent the risk of a repetitive and bland meal plan, you can introduce alternative whole grains like wild rice, millet, and amaranth to your selection. Some supermarkets these days have bulk bins. Bulk bins are a pocket-friendly way to experiment with different grains without spending too much in the process.

• **Poultry, Fish, and Meat** — According to the American Heart Association, two fish servings a week is recommended for a healthy person. Go for lean cuts of meat and skinless poultry, and do not forget portion control. Stay away from processed meats and deli meats because they are full of sodium.

• **Frozen Food** — Frozen vegetables and fruits can be useful during the winter when most of them are out of production. These foods should not have seasoning, salt, or added sugar. Flavor the food on your own when cooking, so you can control the nutritional value.

• **Dairy Products** — Look for non-fat dairy options so that you can get three daily servings. Luckily, there are so many varieties available in both low-fat and non-fat substitutes.

• **Dried and Canned Food** — Remember to read the labels, so you are aware of the sodium content and recommended serving size. Low-sodium foods and no salt added foods are always a great selection. Remember to check the date on the products. While markets try to keep the product safe for consumption, you may occasionally find one or two items on the shelves that are past their expiration date.

Meal Prep Sundays

Eating healthy is difficult for many people, not because they don't know what to cook, but because they don't have the time. With your busy work schedule, it is easier to grab something at a restaurant than go home to cook. Many people also dread having to wash dishes after cooking their food. An easy solution to this is to cook your meals for the week on Sunday and keep them in small containers that are easy to manage during the week. When you get home, all you have to do is pick one, heat it up, and enjoy. Meal prep Sundays have become popular in many households since most people are at home on Sunday and don't have other responsibilities to take care of. Here are some useful tips that will make your meal prep Sundays easy:

- **Grill your Meat** — To prepare for Sunday, fire up the grill or oven and cook a week's worth of chicken, fish or whatever protein you choose all at once. This drastically reduced the amount of time it takes to prepare your meals later in the week.

- **Prep Vegetables** — Clean and chop vegetables in advance. Cook some and leave some fresh so you can use them during the week in salads.

- **Smoothie Packs** — Prepare and freeze smoothie ingredients in small containers, so you don't have sort through them during the week. You can just pick what you need and eat.

- **Pre-Cook Grains** — Pre-cooking grains will make your work easier during the week. Choose as many grain ingredients as you need for the week and pre-cook them. Let them cool down, then transfer them into Ziploc bags and store in the refrigerator. Remember, these should be consumed within four days.

CHAPTER 8

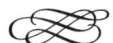

DON'T DRINK YOUR CALORIES

*W*eight gain is a gradual process. Sustainable weight loss should take place gradually, too. A lot of people focus on results instead of the process, and this is one of the reasons why they struggle to find the right approach. If you are result-oriented, you will always end up focusing on options that deliver immediate results, ignoring the risks involved. Processes take time, but they are also effective.

Have you ever wondered why you are not losing weight, even after all the effort you put in? To understand this, you need to think about weight loss as a concept. How does it happen?

For you to lose weight, you should be eating in a calorie deficit. This means you should consume fewer calories than the calories your body burns through physical activity. This deficit should be within a sustainable limit so that your body does not hoard the surplus as fat. At the same time, the deficit should not be insufficient to the point where your body lacks the energy reserves to get you through the day.

From this explanation, if you live an active lifestyle, you

should consume more calories daily compared to a sedentary individual. It is from this concept that fasting and starvation tactics are often proposed. These might work temporarily, but they are not sustainable ideas. Starvation is dangerous. Leave it to celebrities who need to get into a specific shape quickly for a role they are playing. Celebrities work with a lot of well-paid experts to make sure they stay within a healthy limit. You might not have that luxury.

The other challenge with starvation is that you will definitely gain more weight over time. As your body goes into starvation mode, it hoards food and stores it as fat to anticipate lean times ahead.

Instead of going through this experience, it is advisable that you eat the right amount of food daily. Be mindful of your calories so that you oscillate within a healthy range for your weight and your healthy body goals. Weight loss is not just a result of watching your calories; it is the culmination of many other factors, including stress, water retention, a healthy body, and liquid calories. The interesting thing about liquid calories is that they can easily fly under the radar.

Liquid Calories

There is no better definition. Liquid calories are just that, calories in the form of liquids that you consume all the time (Drewnowski & Bellisle, 2007). These calories are present in juice, liquor, milk, soda, and nearly any other drink you consume. Given that these drinks are more of a habitual consumption for most people, you barely think about them in terms of their caloric content.

Let's put it this way – other than water, all drinks contain calories. The drinks you indulge in are made from ingredients that contain calories. Do not assume that liquefaction makes the calories disappear. To understand this better, let's dial back a bit. What are calories?

Calories are a means of estimating the amount of energy

given off by something. As your body digests the food you eat, it burns the food to produce energy. Before you purchase any foods or drinks, read the labels. You will see the amount of energy labeled. The higher the amount on the label, the more energy given off in the course of digestion.

How do we link this to weight loss or gain? Your body burns food to produce energy. You need this energy to power through the day. However, you might not use up all the energy. So, what happens to the surplus energy? Well, magical energy fairies certainly do not make it disappear! Your body keeps it in the form of fat, so it can be used later on. This is how you gain weight.

This also explains why the calorie deficit we mentioned earlier is necessary. When your body is burning calories, it is consuming a lot of energy. Therefore, there is no need to store energy for later use. Essentially, you are not storing fat in your body!

Are calories present in everything? Yes, they are.

When the ingredients are broken down, energy is produced, so everything you consume has calories, including drinks. The challenge with drinks is that you can frequently indulge without even realizing that you have exceeded the limit.

Think about it, how many times have you stopped eating because you felt too full to add another bite, but somehow still had enough room for a few drinks? Drinks are too easy to consume, which creates a problem, especially with weight loss.

Look at it this way, one apple juice serving is around eight ounces, which is roughly a small glass. This serving might have more than a hundred calories. However, if you love your fresh apple juice, and it is easy to access, you will not have only one serving a day. Assuming your consumption is within our threshold, you are consuming an extra 100 calories for every eight ounces you drink. Meanwhile, we have not factored in the other calories you consumed all day through other foods.

One of the biggest challenges with liquid calories is that most of them are obtained from added sugars. Added sugars have zero nutritional value (Park, 2013). We know we should avoid them, but most people never think about the calories in beverages. You might focus on the calorie content of all the foods you eat but ignore the drinks, which creates a bigger problem. Here are some reasons why you need to rethink your liquid calorie consumption:

• **Develop Insulin Resistance** — Your body absorbs these beverages very fast. The challenge here is that your insulin must respond faster so that your blood sugar levels are in check. This works if you consume such drinks occasionally, which most people don't. Persistent consumption of sugary drinks pushes your insulin to work overtime, exhausting your production. It won't be long before you develop insulin resistance. Your hormones become weaker and ineffective over time, but your body needs to find a way to produce more insulin. Insulin resistance marks the onset of many health problems. You will pack weight around your midsection, and if you don't do anything about it, you could develop heart disease, diabetes, infertility, and other health issues.

• **Focus on Nutrient Density** — Remember how you insist on getting value for your money each time you go shopping? Why not do the same with your food? Think about nutrient density (Bohma, 2018). Nutrient density means you focus on foods that contain more nutrients for each calorie you consume. One of the best examples is kale, which is loaded with antioxidants, minerals, fiber, and vitamins. The other challenge with liquid calories is that they do not make you feel full. Instead, you feel hungrier after consuming such liquids, which means you will eat more than you should. Sugary smoothies and fruit juices are notorious for this since they lack the necessary fiber that makes you full.

• **Drink for Weight Loss** — Instead of consuming sugary beverages, consider switching things up with water. Drinks are the easiest way for additional calories to sneak into your body. These are calories you consume without moderation, which eventually get stored as fat. If you are serious about weight loss, drop the habit. Stop drinking anything that contains additional calories. Soda, juices, caffeinated drinks, and sweetened iced tea are some examples of drinks you need to avoid. Apart from that, do not add sweeteners to your drinks. They might taste bland, but your taste buds adapt quickly. Before you know it, you will get used to, and enjoy the changes.

Warning Signs Your Liquid Calories Are Getting out of Hand

Having discussed some of the risks behind liquid calories, how can you tell whether you are on the right track? What is it about your lifestyle that will make you realize you need a reality check? Here are some unhealthy habits that should alert you:

• **Early Morning Smoothies** — Juices and smoothies are some of the biggest fallacies in nutrition. Many people believe they are a healthy option, and for this reason, they are the go-to breakfast recipe, especially for busy professionals. However, some smoothies do the opposite, especially those that you buy from the local fruit juice store or coffee shop (Tallmadge, 2013). Most of these drinks have added fat and sugar to sweeten them. This means that, by the time you are done with your drink, you might have already consumed around half of the calories you need for the rest of the day. Some people believe smoothies are so healthy that they will have more than one drink a day – one in the morning and another later in the afternoon. If you add the food calories, you are doing poorly.

- **Your Love for Cocktails** — Whenever you meet up with your friends, one of the first things you might do is order some fancy cocktails. You don't know which mixer the restaurant uses, so you will be consuming an unknown number of calories with each shot. For those crazy nights when you down an unknown number of cocktails, you can only speculate at the number of calories you consume.

- **Yo-Yo-Type Energy Levels** — Sugary beverages have the uncanny ability to crash your energy throughout the day. Immediately after you finish your drink, you have this amazing sugar rush, and you feel like you can conquer anything that stands in your way. However, a short while later, you are exhausted and don't have the energy to lift a finger. Your best bet is to find a glass of water.

- **Persistent Thirst** — If you are thirsty, drink pure water or other healthy alternatives. Non-water beverages give you the illusion that they quench your thirst, but they can make your situation worse. These drinks raise your blood sugar levels, which explains why you are thirsty all the time. In case you need some flavor in your water, add lime, lemon, or mint.

- **Inaccurate Perception of Liquid Calories** — There is no difference between liquid calories and calories consumed in solid form. Calories are just the same. The misconception that liquid calories are different from solid calories is unfounded and leads many people to consume unnecessary drinks. Most of the fancy drinks you get in the morning on your way to the office are obvious culprits, like frozen coffee drinks and pumpkin spice lattes. These drinks are loaded with full-fat dairy, sugary syrup, and in some cases, whipped cream. Sports drinks are another category you should stay away from, given that they might also include sodium.

- **Belly Fat** — You are keeping a healthy diet, but for some reason, your belly keeps growing. At this juncture, you need to rethink your meals. Investigate what you drink, and you might find the answer. For example, you might drink a soda with most of your meals. Did you know that a can of soda has around 150 calories? This translates to around ten teaspoons of sugar. Avoid these sugary drinks by any means possible.

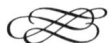

CHAPTER 9

*E*motional eating is a situation where your go-to response for anything that throws you out of your comfort zone is to eat, whether you are hungry or not. Most people who struggle with emotional eating, also known as **emotional hunger**, tend to crave foods rich in carbohydrates and calories, yet these foods have very little nutritional value. These foods are comfort foods. Some of the most notorious comfort foods are:

- Pizza
- French fries
- Chips
- Chocolate
- Cookies
- Ice cream

When dealing with anxiety or stress, many people turn to emotional eating to take their minds away from the issues at hand. There are also those whose response to stress is an inhibited appetite, while a much smaller population does not experience any change in their appetite in such situations. It follows, therefore, that stress is one of the leading factors associated with weight loss and gain.

Emotional eating is also one of the early symptoms that experts look for to indicate atypical depression. However, there are many people who engage in emotional eating but are not clinically depressed. Their predisposition to emotional eating is because of chronic stress or momentary overwhelming feelings (Adriaanse, de Ridder, & Evers, 2010).

We live in a highly competitive world that is advancing at supersonic speed. People are exposed to stressful situations at a very early age. Many people today are forced to mature before they should so that they can take advantage of opportunities that come their way and live better lives. With this in mind, the propensity to develop unhealthy eating habits starts at an early age. If unchecked, this can spiral into a food obsession.

Relationship Between Stress and Body Weight

Why do you retain fat when you are stressed? The answer is in cortisol, the hormone responsible for stress (Young, 2019). In normal situations, your body secretes just the right amount of cortisol. However, when you are stressed, the production goes into overdrive. The production is highest in the mornings and lowest in the evenings.

Imagine a situation where your body is flooded with stress hormones early in the morning when you are supposed to be at your best. This inhibits all activities you will engage in that day because you start the day on the wrong foot. Disrupted cortisol production does not just influence weight gain; it also affects where the additional weight is stashed in your body. Most of the fat you gain during this period is concentrated in your abdominal area.

Are You Dealing with Binge Eating or Emotional Eating?

Binge eating and emotional eating are two concepts that

are closely related. The main difference between them is in the amount of food you eat. In both of these scenarios, you have a difficult time controlling your cravings. However, in emotional eating, you consume moderate or large amounts of food.

Binge eating, on the other hand, is an eating disorder on its own and is often accompanied by purging afterward. It is a disorder where you are continually overeating out of compulsion. Binge eaters consume more food than the average person would within a given period of time, even if they are not hungry. A binge eater will try to hide the truth about how much food they consume, because they are ashamed of it. When eating together with other people, they might also eat faster than everyone else.

Why Do You Resort to Food?

Negative emotions create an emotional void, a sense of emptiness in your mind. When this happens, most people resort to food because the satiety makes them feel whole again, albeit for a short time. Once again, we must recognize the role that your mind plays in this predicament. You do not feel hungry. You find yourself in a situation that requires emotional intelligence, yet your subconscious mind pushes you towards food.

There are many other things that might be responsible for this predicament, including the following:

• **Inactive Lifestyle** — If you are generally inactive, you will struggle to manage stress effectively. There are many simple activities that can help you relieve stress. Going outside for a walk might seem like a mundane activity, but the impact in stress management is profound. How about going to the gym, jogging, cycling, or taking your pets out for a walk? All of these are activities that you might take for granted, but they can help you overcome stress. People who are inactive and do not engage in any of these or similar activities will often lack an avenue to release stress, and easily turn to food.

- **Lack of Support Network** — What does your social circle look like? Your support network comes in handy at your time of emotional need. You need people around you who will assure you that everything is okay, and it is normal to go through what you are experiencing. Without this network, you are all alone, boxed into a corner. Life can take a toll on you. If you cannot find someone to talk to about what you are going through, you might feel desperate to get home, lock the door, slump onto the couch, and devour a bowl of ice cream, alone. This is common for people who withdraw from or cannot receive social support during a time of emotional upheaval.

- **Inaccurate Interpretation of Hunger** — How well do you understand your hunger pangs? Unbeknownst to most people, there is a difference between emotional hunger and physical hunger. If you cannot tell the two apart, you will always find something to eat to satisfy either of them. What is the difference? Physical hunger is a gradual process. Your hunger pangs will grow slowly to a point where you cannot hold on any longer. To satisfy physical hunger, virtually any food will do. When you find food, you stop eating the moment you are satisfied and feel full, during which time you will not feel bad about satisfying your cravings. Now, the difference between this and satisfying emotional hunger is that emotional hunger does not grow gradually. It creeps up on you suddenly. With emotional hunger, your cravings are for specific foods. You can keep eating until you feel physically full, but this will still not satisfy you. In the end, you feel ashamed or guilty about overindulging. One of the challenges when dealing with emotional eating is that you often feel powerless about your inability to control your emotions, not emotional eating. This explains why most people feel guilty after they have consumed a lot of food.

- **Altered Cortisol Levels** — The drastic change in cortisol levels in your body in response to stress can lead to cravings. Stress eating is one of the reasons why most people fail to meet their weight goals. The best way to beat this is to find ways of relieving stress without overeating. Stress can slow down or impede your appetite. When facing undue pressure, your nervous system signals the adrenal glands to produce epinephrine (adrenaline). In this state, your body temporarily halts your appetite. If you overcome the situation, all systems resume normal functionality. Not everyone is that lucky. At times, stress persists. If this happens, the adrenal glands produce cortisol. Cortisol does not just increase your appetite; it also heightens your motivation, including your desire to eat. The level of cortisol in the bloodstream will increase until you overcome the stressful episode. After that, it falls. If you do not overcome the stressful incident, the body will still produce more cortisol, leaving you vulnerable to overeating. Sugary foods dampen stress impulses, emotions, and responses. This is why they are referred to as comfort foods. They make you feel comfortable in the knowledge that they counteract stress. If you do it once and it works, your subconscious believes that this is the best solution, and it becomes your go-to move whenever you are stressed.
- **Negative Self-Talk** — Granted, everyone goes through periods of uncertainty and stress from time to time. How you manage them can make a big difference. In these situations, some people embrace negative self-talk (Talmay, 2014). This is an unhealthy habit that can result in unhealthy eating. Food offers a distraction. Instead of dealing with the emotional upheaval, you eat and pretend you are okay. The problem here is that you must still face your fears at some

point. You have to deal with the situation. The happiness and relief you feel once you indulge in comfort foods is only temporary.

Factors That Encourage Emotional Eating

If you get to a point where your response to emotional upheaval is to eat, you will struggle with emotional eating. There are many reasons why you might be struggling with emotional eating. Here are some of the possible reasons for your challenges and simple solutions:

• **Unconscious Indulgence** — One of the reasons behind emotional eating is that you are not paying attention to the food you eat or why you eat it. You don't know the triggers to look out for (Rogers, 2016). Unconscious eating, or eating without paying attention, is a situation where you keep on eating even when you are full. You can do this even when you planned to stop eating and pack the rest of the food away. The solution here is to learn how to be mindful of what you are eating and when you are eating. It might not be easy at the beginning, but you will get the hang of it later on. You will also learn how to conquer self-pity and judgment, and feel better without using food as an outlet.

• **Limited Pleasure Outlets** — Many people have nothing else they enjoy beyond food. They don't have an activity they can indulge in out of pleasure. When they have cravings, the only solution is to look for comfort food. This is an unhealthy habit. Most comfort foods are loaded with a lot of sugar. The problem with too much sugar is that it releases opioids in the brain. Opioids are the key ingredients present in heroin, cocaine, and many other narcotic substances. What this teaches us is that the calming sensation you get from comfort food is real, though it will not last. Dropping emotional eating, therefore, might be as difficult as dropping a drug habit. Think of other reward mechanisms other than eating to excess or any destructive behavior. At first, they might not be as soothing as the food was, but if you give them time, they will be.

• **Managing Difficult Feelings** — From a young age, you learn to run away from bad things. Your brain learns that anything that is not good for you has no room in your life. In some cases, it is better to confront the bad things instead of running away. To deal with such moments, some people find comfort food convenient, hence increasing their suscepti-bility to emotional eating. It is not easy to unlearn things that you have held onto for many years, but it is not impossible either. Don't shy away from a difficult situation. Confront it, and embrace the sadness, rejection, and other feelings that come with it. It might not change your situation, but it builds your endurance.

• **Physiological Challenges** — Going hungry for a long time or exerting yourself too much can pave the way for emotional eating. When you are famished, your desire is to eat the first thing you come across. You don't care what you eat, as long as the rumbling in your stomach stops. In such situations, you set yourself up for failure. It is almost impos-sible to fight off urges and cravings. If you are tired, get some sleep. The solution to hunger is to eat small meals during the day. If you are constantly eating, it is highly unlikely that you will feel the need to overeat. Besides, you can also turn away some food if you still feel full.

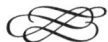

CHAPTER 10

EXERCISING

The decision to start working out is a bold one. Many people think about it but never go all the way, so congratulations! This is the first step of many that will result in you living a healthy and satisfying life. Working out is not just about the exercise routines you perform; it is also about improving your mind, body and spirit.

Beginner's Guide to Exercise

From a beginner's perspective, it is always best to start small and make gradual progress over time. The benefits of exercise have long been documented, so take pride in the fact that you are on the right path. You have many options for working out. As long as you do it right, you can reap amazing rewards from different levels and types of exercise.

In respect to weight loss, any physical exercise counts towards your overall goals, and you feel better afterward. Exercise is good for your moods, too. Your options are endless and include anything from riding a bike, walking, dancing, or even doing your household chores. The underlying factor is that you should enjoy whichever activity you choose to engage in.

The American Heart Association recommends at least half an hour of exercise daily (Pina, et al., 2003). During this period, you should engage in moderate or intense physical activities. This is enough to keep you healthy. However, even if you are getting ten minutes of regular exercise daily, you will still reap benefits, and ten minutes is better than none. The goal here is to encourage you to live an active lifestyle.

When is the Best Time to Exercise?

When you are trying to build a habit of exercise, it is important to plan around what works best for your schedule. There is mixed evidence on what time of day is ideal for exercising. Exercising in the morning or waiting until the evenings both offer their own benefits. It largely comes down to what works best with your schedule. However, new research is surfacing that indicates morning workout routines are potentially the most effective for long-term success.

Professor of psychiatry and human behavior Dale Bond, Ph.D., of the Brown Alpert Medical School created a study that reveals a link between the time of a day that a person exercises and their ability to keep up a consistent workout routine. His survey of 375 adults who had maintained at least 30 pounds of weight loss for a full year revealed two things about people with solid exercise routines (at least 2 days per week in this study). First, 68 percent of those subjects typically worked out at the same time each day. Second, nearly half (47.8 percent) of the people who had consistent routines worked out in the early morning instead of the late morning, afternoon, or evening.

Preparation

Before you begin any routine, you must prepare adequately. One of the first things to do is check to make sure you are healthy enough for what lies ahead. Are you fit enough to perform the activities you plan on doing? See your doctor and discuss what your plans are. This is especially directed to those who are 45 years old and older. There are major health risks as you grow older, which might be exacerbated by exercise, or make it impossible for you to achieve your fitness goals.

One thing that is certain is that, regardless of whatever medical condition you might be suffering from, there is almost always something you can do to work out. Talk to an expert about this. There are workout regimes for virtually any medical issue, so you just need to find the right exercise for you.

Why should you get medical clearance before you start? Other than ensuring you are healthy and fit for the rigors that lie ahead, medical clearance also helps you plan for your fitness goals. From that assessment, you can know whether you are capable of running in the next 5K marathon, or if you are ready to start intense workout sessions at the gym, and so forth.

The main idea when working out is to start slow and improve gradually. Remember that your body also needs enough time to recover. One of the mistakes that many beginners make is to hit their fitness routine with insane aggression. You will burn out very fast. There is also a higher risk that you will get injured. Recovery the next day can be very difficult, and some people never resume their fitness plans again after experiencing the recovery pain and soreness. Aggressive beginners never make it all the way. They quit as soon as they realize that things are difficult. If you start slow and work your way up, your body adapts to the pressure with each step-up, which makes it easier for you to keep working out.

Frequently Used Fitness Terms

There are some terms that you will come across often as you work out. Understanding them gives you a deeper knowledge of what you are working on, and what you stand to gain from it. Let's take a look at some of them:

1. **Maximum Heart Rate** — This rate depends on your age. It is derived by subtracting your age from 220.

2. **Cardiovascular Activity (Aerobics)** — Aerobic activities are routines that are intense enough to speed up your heart rate and your breathing. Some examples include swimming, running, dancing, and cycling.

3. **Stretching (Flexibility Training)** — Stretching helps to widen the motion range of your joints. As you grow older, your tendons, muscles, and ligaments tighten and become shorter. It is easy to confuse stretching and warming up, but they are not the same thing. Never make the mistake of stretching cold joints and muscles. You increase the risk of injury if you do this. Warm up first.

4. **Warm Up** — This is a process where you get your body ready for exercise. Exercise exerts pressure and stress on different parts of your body. Light aerobic movements like brisk walking and jogging help warm you up. The idea behind warming up is to make your blood circulation more efficient during the workouts. As the blood flow increases, the resulting heat warms your joints and muscles. It is wise to follow a warm up with some stretches.

5. **Resistance Training** — This training involves weight and strength training. The idea is to make you stronger and improve muscle functions. There are unique exercises that target different muscle groups.

6. **Sets** — A set is a loose reference in resistance training where you repeat a specific routine a number of times. For example, you can perform 10 sit-ups, rest a bit then perform another set of 10 sit-ups.

7. **Repetition** — This refers to the number of times you perform a specific activity in a set.

8. **Cooldown** — Just like you warmed up before your

workout, you need to cool down, too. Cooldowns are exercise sets that are not strenuous. They are performed at the end of an intense workout. An example is if you were running on the treadmill. A cooldown session would involve slowing down the speed so you can walk until your heart rate returns to its normal level.

Exercise without Going to the Gym

You do not necessarily need to go to the gym to work out. There is so much that you can do on your own in the comfort of your house. Simple routines like sit-ups, pushups, and lunges allow you to use the weight of your body for resistance training (Kamb, 2013). However, just because you do not need a gym does not mean you cannot create something like it at home. Some of the equipment today is affordable, and you can create your own workout space at home. You can buy the following:

- Free Weights
- Treadmill
- Exercise ball
- Workout DVDs and online videos
- Weight stacks, flexible rods, and bands

Gym equipment and environments can be overrated. Most gym facilities strive to get memberships at any cost. As a result, they use different promotional techniques to lure you in. Many customers join gyms without a clear plan, and they quit shortly after when they realize the process is not sustainable. This happens a lot at the beginning of the year when people are making resolutions they hope to keep.

While going to the gym has its perks, there are challenges, too. It is expensive. Most of the best gyms wherever you live will cost a pretty penny. This explains why, even if they are committed, most people do not last more than two or three months. If the idea of a gym is out of the question for you, let's look at some techniques you can use to enhance your fitness goals without a gym membership:

- **Keep Walking** — While walking might not be as intense as running, it has its own benefits, and is good for your heart. Local walking clubs have become popular over the years, so find one with people you can interact with. Such individuals will motivate you to keep coming back. If you don't have a local walking club, start one. You can start with your friends and family members. When you get to the office, get up from your desk and walk around the office. Instead of sitting down all the time, occasionally work from your computer while standing, so that your body can stretch. Over the weekends and holidays, you can take long walks, especially if you live by the beach.

- **Running** — You burn a lot of calories while running. This is an activity you can perform wherever you are. You also strengthen your leg muscles while at it. Many local parks today have jogging trails. Some institutions also allow the public free access to their facilities at specific times. If your schedule allows, and you live in a safe place, run a few miles in the morning before you go to work. Exercising early in the morning can give you a nice boost of energy that lasts the whole day. Plus, if you wait until the end of the day, there is always the risk that you might be too tired to keep up with your exercise routine.

- **Visit Local Recreation Centers** — Local recreation centers are made available by the local administration. Their registration fees are affordable, and in some cases, you have free access. These centers may also have running trails, indoor pools, some workout equipment, and more. Some enterprising individuals also offer workout training at the centers for a fee. If your local gym is too expensive, look for a YMCA in the neighborhood. They always have awesome facilities.

- **Join an Amateur Sports Team** — Amateur sports teams are free to join, or are accessible for a modest fee. Once you find a group that is committed to playing a game for fun, this can be your fitness plan. In some cases, the amateur teams go on to participate in local tournaments, but essentially the idea is to have fun and stay fit.

- **Use Public Courts** — Many public courts have volleyball, tennis, basketball, and other activities that you can participate in during your free time. While you might be required to bring your equipment, the courts are usually free. This is a good way to exercise with your loved ones, and probably meet other like-minded individuals in the process.

- **Buy Your Exercise Equipment** — Who needs a gym membership when you can get equipment cheaply? One of the best activities you can perform at home is indoor cycling. Owning a stationary bike means that you can use it even when it is raining outside, or when you feel you don't have enough time for a proper workout. Most of the equipment you can use at home is foldable and can be stored easily, so you don't have to worry about space.

- **Watch Online Exercise Videos** — From yoga to high-intensity interval training, today, you can access different video tutorials online on YouTube or from the website of the trainer. The videos show how to perform some routines step-by-step, which you can do at home. Such resources work, but you must be motivated and committed to working out. Many people are not disciplined enough, and they quit as soon as their schedule gets complicated, or they start procrastinating. The videos are perfect in the morning to help you supercharge your day.

- **Find a Swimming Pool** — Swimming is a fantastic full-body fitness routine that doesn't damage your joints. Community pools will come in handy in case you don't have one at home. Other than swimming, you can also join a deep-water aerobics class.

- **Cycling** — If you are running quick errands, get a bicycle instead of driving. Cycling will help you burn a lot of calories. Bicycles are easy to carry, so you can lift it over your shoulder and jog a bit as part of your resistance training. If you live close to your place of work, cycle to work instead of getting that bus ride.

- **Play with Your Pets and Children** — Young children are always buzzing with energy. Spending time with them or your pets when you get home from work is one of the most enthralling activities you can perform, which will help you stay fit. If you have a very playful pet, you can get as much of a workout as possible from an hour playing together. Besides, the activities you engage in with your children and pets are more satisfying than anything you might do on a treadmill.

All the options we have discussed are either free or affordable. You don't need to sign up for a gym membership when you can stay fit from the comfort of your home. Try to make your routines fun so that you look forward to them. This is an easy way to stay motivated and work towards your weight loss goals.

Always Take the Stairs

Skip the elevator and take the stairs. This is such a simple activity that can yield significant benefits for your health. Taking the stairs will go a long way and help you improve your fitness levels. If you live or work in a high-rise building, this can be a very good fitness routine.

Like most fitness routines, use the stairs gradually. You will not just wake up one day and climb thirty floors. Start with a few flights, then take the elevator the rest of the way. Add a few flights of stairs as you get used to the exercise. After a while, you will have a system in place.

Do not underestimate the power of climbing stairs. This is also an activity about which you must consult your doctor before you begin. Individuals who have pre-existing conditions or injuries, particularly in the legs and knees, should not try this unless your doctor advises you otherwise. Regarding your fitness goals, here are some benefits of using the stairs frequently:

• **Effortless Workout** — Taking the stairs is one of the most efficient workout routines. A simple commute could easily turn into a fitness routine that helps you burn calories. The effort you need to climb up a flight of stairs can also help you reap benefits similar to a cardio session at the gym.

• **Strengthens Your Heart** — Aerobic exercises strengthen your heart. This is what you can expect when you take the stairs. You don't need to hit the road running or go to the gym and sweat it out. Using the stairs is a simple routine that works out your heart and muscles, especially your leg and core muscles. The more you climb stairs and make it a routine, the easier it will be for you to manage your sleep, weight, stress hormones, cholesterol, and blood sugar levels. Using the stairs is a good way to supercharge your metabolism, and it also promotes healthy bones.

• **Mental Empowerment** — Like any other exercise, taking the stairs is about more than physical benefits. There are mental benefits, too. These workout routines improve your attitude and help you reduce your stress levels.

• **Stronger Legs** — Using the stairs puts pressure on the muscle groups around your legs. Strengthening these muscles helps your balance and posture. It also helps in toning your calves, butt, and thighs. Use the stairs as often as you can to help stabilize your knees and ankles.

• **Easy Milestones** — It is always advisable that you start working out slowly and build on your progress gradually. This is something that you can do easily when you take the stairs. If you climb two flights of stairs this week, next week you increase it to four flights, and so on. You could also try increasing your speed of going up the stairs while keeping the number of flights unchanged. This will help you burn more calories, too.

You don't have to get to the stair level to begin your workout session. You can start from the moment you get out of your car. When possible, use the parking spot that is furthest away from the office, so that you have enough time to walk and prepare for the flights of stairs.

CONCLUSION

When you started this journey, you might have been conflicted about diets. Diets are no different from political promotional campaigns. They promise you so much so you can get on board. It's true that they can work, but only in the short-term. Soon after, you find yourself right back to where you started, and in many cases, even worse off. Weight loss is not something you should attempt with a short-term perspective. This is about your health and your life. The only way to approach weight loss is with a mindset towards long-term sustainability and results that will last for years.

If you move away from diets, you will realize that there is so much you can do about your weight, and most of the changes you make towards your weight goals will not cost you a thing. At the beginning of this book, we mentioned that diets are not all there is to weight loss. You have probably tried quite a few diets and realized this. Most diets are impractical since they rely on denying your body of some important nutrients. You cannot do that for the long-term. At some point, you will fall back into your old habits, and the weight will come back like you had never lost it in the first place.

The answers you seek in weight loss diets lie within your subconscious. Your mind creates a perception of your ideal weight, and you take it as the gospel truth. By challenging these core beliefs, you make vital steps towards realizing your weight loss objectives. You must embrace behavioral changes to achieve the desired results. Without changing your mind, you will do the same things you have always done and get the same results.

Stay away from people who limit your beliefs about yourself or your weight. Constantly bombarding your mind with such messages can turn you into a negative person. You must challenge yourself to be better than what you think you are. It is only when you change your actions and beliefs that you can come closer to realizing your weight loss objectives.

The best way to go about weight loss is to make it a habitual process. Humans are creatures of habit. When we find something we like, we get used to it. There are small, healthy habits that you can introduce into your daily routine that will encourage you to stay fit and lose weight in the process. These are activities you can regularly perform without interfering with your normal schedule. Such habits encourage you to follow a routine and learn the importance of discipline in the process.

You have so much more control over your life than you realize. You have the power to change your environment and the activities in your environment. You need an enabling environment to achieve your weight loss objectives in the same way you need an enabling environment to succeed at work. Look at your pantry, for example. If you have junk food in the house, you will eat it. If you replace it with healthier alternatives, you are much more likely to eat healthy. By the end of the day, everything in your kitchen is there because you made a conscious decision to buy it.

Choices come with consequences. In terms of weight loss, every decision you make either comes back to haunt you, or works in your favor. Today, we eat more food than we used to a few decades back. This is a huge societal concern. Portions have grown larger over the years. Large portions create a problem for you when you are working to lose weight. Luckily for you, it is not mandatory that you must clear your plate. We discussed some useful tips for portion control that will help you avoid overeating. Once you are aware of how much food is enough for you, you can take preventive measures to avoid binge eating or eating to excess, even when you are eating out at restaurants.

Your meal plans play an important role in determining your weight loss success. Take a look at your shopping list and rethink your choices. There are lots of healthy options out there, and most of them are affordable. Take vegetables, for example. We have different varieties in the market. Every time you go shopping, try out something new. Most people do not eat as many vegetables and fruits as they should. Get into a habit of having some vegetables with your meals, even if it's just a few slices or pieces. It grows on you, and before you know it, you love the outcome. Besides, vegetables do not have a lot of calories, so you can usually eat as many as you want without affecting your calorie deficit.

Emotional eating is your worst enemy when it comes to weight loss. Eating to satisfy cravings leads you down a rabbit hole that you may never get out of. To stop this habit, you must learn the difference between emotional hunger and real hunger. The secret here is to listen to your body. Pay attention to the hunger triggers, so you know the difference between these two. Rising above emotional eating is about being mindful of what you eat, and, more importantly, being mindful of what your body needs.

The most important takeaway from this book is activity. You have to be active to achieve your weight loss objectives. People have different activity levels. Being active does not necessarily mean you must enroll in a gym. If you can, and you find that it works for you, then, by all means, continue! However, there are easier and more affordable options all around you. If you stop for a minute and look around you after reading this book, you will realize how lucky you are. Everything you need to help you work out is within your reach. Take the stairs, spare half an hour and run in the morning, join your local amateur team, go swimming, or play with your children. All of these are things that help you stay fit.

Weight loss is about commitment. You commit to this for the long-term. You lay out your goals and a roadmap for success, and you work towards it every single day. This is not a sprint; it is a marathon. Resist the urge to go after quick fixes, and instead, embrace gradual changes. It might take time before you drop some pounds, but rest assured that when you do, they will not come back to bite you.

Ideally, you need to focus on three things: increasing your activity level, eating healthy, and changing your mindset. If you conquer these three things, nothing will stand in your way. You have to change the way you think about weight, the food you eat, your activities, and yourself. Stop buying unhealthy food. Read food labels, so you understand what you are putting into your body. More importantly, don't stop moving.

You are in control. You've got this!

REFERENCES

Aamodt, S. (2013, June). Why dieting doesn't usually work. Retrieved from https://www.ted.com/talks/sandra_aamod-t_why_dieting_doesn_t_usually_work

Adriaanse, M. A., de Ridder, D. T., & Evers, C. (2010). Emotional eating: Eating when emotional or emotional about eating? *Psychology & Health,26*(1), 23-39. doi:10.1080/08870440903207627

American Heart Association. (2018, March 6). Understanding Food Nutrition Labels. Retrieved from https://www.heart.org/en/healthy-living/healthy-eating/eat-smart/ nutrition-basics/understanding-food-nutrition-labels

Bertelli, A. M., & Carson, J. L. (2011). Small changes, big results: Legislative voting behavior in the presence of new voters. *Electoral Studies,30*(1), 201-209. doi:10.1016/j.elect-stud.2011.01.002

Boham, E. (2018, March 05). Stop Drinking Your Calories! Retrieved from https://www.ultrawellnesscenter.-com/2018/03/05/stop-drinking-calories/

Bokhari, D. (n.d.). The Power of Habit: 3 Steps To

Creating Good Habits (and Breaking Bad Habits). Retrieved from https://www.meaningfulhq.com/the-power-of-habit.html

Charles Duhigg's 'The Power of Habit' - 13 Key Insights. (2015, November 21). Retrieved from https://heleo.com/13-key-insights-charles-duhiggs-power-habit/2026/

Clear, J. (2018, October 24). How to Build New Habits: This is Your Strategy Guide. Retrieved from https://jamesclear.com/habit-guide

Considine, R. V. (2003). Endocrine Regulation of Leptin Production. *Leptin and Reproduction,39*-51. doi:10.1007/978-1-4615-0157-2_3

Desbordes, G. (2016). On the Relationship Between Mindfulness and Buddhism (Hint: It's Complicated). *PsycCRITIQUES,6161*(2323). doi:10.1037/a0040339

Drewnowski, A., & Bellisle, F. (2007). Liquid calories, sugar, and body weight. *The American Journal of Clinical Nutrition,85*(3), 651-661. doi:10.1093/ajcn/85.3.651

Edison, T. A. (1900). U.S. patents issued to Thomas A. Edison from 1883-88. doi:10.5479/sil.472335.39088007608003

Feinle-Bisset, C., Patterson, M., Ghatei, M. A., Bloom, S. R., & Horowitz, M. (2005). Fat digestion is required for suppression of ghrelin and stimulation of peptide YY and pancreatic polypeptide secretion by intraduodenal lipid. *American Journal of Physiology-Endocrinology and Metabolism,289*(6). doi:10.1152/ajpendo.00220.2005

Galante, J., Iribarren, S. J., & Pearce, P. F. (2012). Effects of mindfulness-based cognitive therapy on mental disorders: A systematic review and meta-analysis of randomised controlled trials. *Journal of Research in Nursing,18*(2), 133-155. doi:10.1177/1744987112466087

Gao, L., Li, Y., Fei, D., Ma, L., Chen, S., Feng, B., . . . Ji, L. (2017). Prevalence of and risk factors for diabetic ketosis in

Chinese diabetic patients with random blood glucose levels 13.9 mmol/L: Results from the China study in prevalence of diabetic ketosis (CHECK) study. *Journal of Diabetes, 10*(3), 249-255. doi:10.1111/1753-0407.12582

Goldstein, C. M., Thomas, J. G., Wing, R. R., & Bond, D. S. (2017). Successful weight loss maintainers use health-tracking smartphone applications more than a nationally representative sample: Comparison of the National Weight Control Registry to Pew Tracking for Health. *Obesity Science & Practice, 3*(2), 117-126. doi:10.1002/osp4.102

Gottlieb, S. (2003). Men should eat nine servings of fruit and vegetables a day. *Bmj, 326*(7397). doi:10.1136/bmj.326.7397.1003/a

Grady, D. (2004, September 11). Unblame the victim: Heart disease causes vary. Retrieved from http://www.ncbi.nlm.nih.gov/pubmed/15487058

Gunnars, K. (2018, March 14). How to Lose Weight Fast: 3 Simple Steps, Based on Science. Retrieved from https://www.healthline.com/nutrition/how-to-lose-weight-as-fast-as-possible

Hathaway, M. D. (2017). Overcoming Fear, Denial, Myopia, and Paralysis. *Worldviews, 21*(2), 175-193. doi:10.1163/15685357-02002100

Hildrew, C. (2018). Growth mindset for students and families. *Becoming a Growth Mindset School,* 135-144. doi:10.4324/9781315179506-12

Hook, D. B. (2009, August 05). How Portion Size Adds Up to Obesity. Retrieved from https://www.everydayhealth.com/diet-nutrition/weight-management/big-food-are-we-eating-more.aspx

Issler, K. D. (2009). Inner Core Belief Formation, Spiritual Practices, and the Willing-Doing Gap. *Journal of Spiritual Formation and Soul Care, 2*(2), 179-198. doi:10.1177/193979090900200203

Jacka, F. N., & Berk, M. (2013, September 16). Depression, diet and exercise. Retrieved from http://www.ncbi.nlm.nih.gov/pubmed/25370279

Kamb, S. (2013). 40 Ways to Exercise without Realizing It. Retrieved from https://www.nerdfitness.com/blog/25-ways-to-exercise-without-realizing-it/

Kim, J. W. (2015). Reid on Particularism, Habit, and Personal Identity. *Journal of Scottish Philosophy,13*(3), 203-217. doi:10.3366/jsp.2015.0104

Lawrence, W. (1993, July). The Commission on Cancer and the American Cancer Society: Partners in cancer control. Retrieved from http://www.ncbi.nlm.nih.-gov/pubmed/10127226

Masuda, A., & Hill, M. L. (2013). Mindfulness as therapy for disordered eating: A systematic review. *Neuropsychiatry,3*(4), 433-447. doi:10.2217/npy.13.36

Nöth, W. (2016). Habits, Habit Change, and the Habit of Habit Change According to Peirce. *Studies in Applied Philosophy, Epistemology and Rational Ethics Consensus on Peirce's Concept of Habit,*35-63. doi:10.1007/978-3-319-45920-2_3

Oppong, T. (2018, August 21). How to Instantly Reframe Your Mindset And Radically Improve Your Life. Retrieved from https://medium.com/thrive-global/how-to- instantly-reframe-your-mindset-and-radically-improve-your-life-d12afa6fbd67

Orbell, S., & Verplanken, B. (2010). The automatic component of habit in health behavior: Habit as cue-contingent automaticity. *Health Psychology,29*(4), 374-383. doi:10.1037/a0019596

Park, S. (2013). Removing dietary liquid calories prevents accelerated body mass index increase. *The Journal of Pediatrics,162*(3), 655. doi:10.1016/j.jpeds.2012.12.090

Piña, I. L., Apstein, C. S., Balady, G. J., Belardinelli, R., Chaitman, B. R., Duscha, B. D., . . . Sullivan, M. J. (2003).

Exercise and Heart Failure. *Circulation, 107*(8), 1210-1225. doi:10.1161/01.cir.0000055013.92097.40

Pluchevskaya, E. (2017). Application of the SWOT-analysis as an evaluation tool to achieve state of personal well-being. doi:10.15405/epsbs.2017.01.74

Purdy, C. (2019, February 28). Fast food portion sizes, calories, and sodium are all rising. Retrieved from https://qz.com/1562476/fast-food-portion-sizes-calories-and-sodium-are-all-rising/

Rogers, M. (2016, February 27). 7 Ways To Banish Emotional Eating For Good. Retrieved from https://www.-mindbodygreen.com/0-23917/7-ways-to-banish-emotional-eating-for-good.html

Schultz, M. B. (2017). Conceptual Congruence in Mindfulness-Based Weight Loss Intervention Studies. *Mindfulness, 9*(4), 1028-1036. doi:10.1007/s12671-017-0860-5

Scott, S. J. (2019, March 28). Best Portion Control Tips: 11 Ways to Avoid Portion Distortion. Retrieved from https://www.developgoodhabits.com/portion- control-tips/

Selig, M. (2010, October 21). Why Diets Don't Work...And What Does. Retrieved from https://www.psychologytoday.com/us/blog/changepower/201010/why-diets-dont-workand-what-does

Soederberg Miller, L. M. (2016). Nutrition Label Literacy. *AADE in Practice, 4*(4), 38-42. doi:10.1177/2325160316650253

Son, Y., & Kim, G. (2012). The Relationship between Obesity, Self-esteem and Depressive Symptoms of Adult Women in Korea. *The Korean Journal of Obesity, 21*(2), 89. doi:10.7570/kjo.2012.21.2.89

Strohacker, K., Carpenter, K. C., & McFarlin, B. K. (n.d.). Consequences of Weight Cycling: An Increase in Disease Risk? Retrieved from http://www.ncbi.nlm.nih.gov/pubmed/25429313

Tallmadge, K. (2013, August 06). Stealth Assault on Health: Beverages Pack Calorie Punch (Op-Ed). Retrieved from https://www.livescience.com/38694-keeping- calories-from-juice-in-check.html

Talmay, O. (2014, June 11). Conquer Emotional Eating With These 12 Weird Tricks. Retrieved from https://www.huffpost.com/entry/conquer-emotional-eating- with-these-12-weird-tricks_b_5471268

Tamarkin, S. (2018, July 28). 13 Experts On Why They No Longer Recommend Diets. Retrieved from https://www.buzzfeed.com/sallytamarkin/weight-neutral-dietitians

Thum, M. (2012, November 26). The Right Mindset: Change Your Mindset in 6 Steps. Retrieved from https://www.myrkothum.com/mindset/

Verplanken, B., & Aarts, H. (1999). Habit, Attitude, and Planned Behaviour: Is Habit an Empty Construct or an Interesting Case of Goal-directed Automaticity? *European Review of Social Psychology, 10*(1), 101-134. doi:10.1080/14792779943000035

Young, R. D. (2019, May 01). 12 Step Program To Conquer Emotional Eating - Once And For All! Retrieved from https://www.bodybuilding.com/fun/12-step-program-to- conquer-emotional-eating-once-and-for-all.htm

Young, S. H. (2018, January 30). 18 Tricks to Make New Habits Stick. Retrieved from https://www.lifehack.org/arti-cles/featured/18-tricks-to-make-new-habits-stick.html

Zuraikat, F. M., Roe, L. S., Sanchez, C. E., & Rolls, B. J. (2018). Comparing the portion size effect in women with and without extended training in portion control: A follow-up to the Portion-Control Strategies Trial. *Appetite, 123*, 334-342. doi:10.1016/j.appet.2018.01.012

Printed in Great Britain
by Amazon

33780628R00071